ACADEMIC PRESS RAPID MANUSCRIPT REPRODUCTION

*Proceedings of a Symposium
on the Physiology and Pathology of Human Aging
Held in Miami, Florida
February 6-7, 1975*

The Physiology and Pathology of Human Aging

Edited by

Ralph Goldman

*Department of Medicine
University of California, Los Angeles
School of Medicine, Los Angeles California*

Morris Rockstein

*Department of Physiology and Biophysics
University of Miami School of Medicine
Miami, Florida*

Associate Editor
Marvin L. Sussman

*Department of Physiology and Biophysics
University of Miami School of Medicine
Miami, Florida*

ACADEMIC PRESS INC., New York San Francisco London 1975
A Subsidiary of Harcourt Brace Jovanovich, Publishers

COPYRIGHT © 1975, BY ACADEMIC PRESS, INC.
ALL RIGHTS RESERVED.
NO PART OF THIS PUBLICATION MAY BE REPRODUCED OR
TRANSMITTED IN ANY FORM OR BY ANY MEANS, ELECTRONIC
OR MECHANICAL, INCLUDING PHOTOCOPY, RECORDING, OR ANY
INFORMATION STORAGE AND RETRIEVAL SYSTEM, WITHOUT
PERMISSION IN WRITING FROM THE PUBLISHER.

ACADEMIC PRESS, INC.
111 Fifth Avenue, New York, New York 10003

United Kingdom Edition published by
ACADEMIC PRESS, INC. (LONDON) LTD.
24/28 Oval Road, London NW1

Library of Congress Cataloging in Publication Data

Symposium on the Physiology and Pathology of Human Aging,
    Miami, Fla., 1975.
    The physiology and pathology of human aging.

    Bibliography: p.
    Includes index.
    1. Geriatrics–Congresses.   2. Aging–Congresses.
I. Goldman, Ralph.   II. Rockstein, Morris.   III. Sussman, Marvin L.   IV. Title.   [DNLM: 1. Aging–Congresses.
WT104 S973p 1975]
RC952.A1S9 1975   618.9'7'07   75-13082
ISBN 0–12–288150–8

PRINTED IN THE UNITED STATES OF AMERICA

CONTENTS

CONTRIBUTORS vii
PREFACE ix
ACKNOWLEDGMENTS xi

The Biology of Aging in Humans—An Overview 1
   Morris Rockstein

Chronologic vs. Biologic Age in Geriatric Patients 9
   Bernard S. Linn

Age Changes in Renal Function 19
   Robert D. Lindeman

Bone-Loss and Aging 39
   Stanley M. Garn

Effects of Human Aging on Drug Absorption and Metabolism 59
   David P. Richey

Biophysical Aspects of Red Cell Aging 95
   David Danon

Cardiac Changes with Age 109
   Raymond Harris

Athero-Arteriosclerosis as an Aging Phenomenon 123
   Herman T. Blumenthal

Memory and Aging 149
   Alvin I. Goldfarb

Aging and Sleep 187
   Joyce D. Kales

Sexual Inadequacy in the Elderly 203
   Ruth B. Weg

Epilogue 229
   Ralph Goldman

CONTRIBUTORS

Herman T. Blumenthal, Aging and Development Program, Department of Psychology, Washington University, St. Louis, Missouri 63130

David Danon, Section of Biological Ultrastructure, The Weizmann Institute of Science, Rehovot, Israel

Stanley M. Garn, Center for Human Growth and Development, The University of Michigan, Ann Arbor, Michigan 48104

Alvin I. Goldfarb, 7 West 96th Street, New York, New York 10025

Ralph Goldman, Department of Medicine, University of California, Los Angeles, School of Medicine, Los Angeles, California 90024

Raymond Harris, Department of Medicine, Albany Medical College, and, Subdepartment of Cardiovascular Medicine, St. Peter's Hospital, Albany, New York 12208

Joyce D. Kales, Sleep Research and Treatment Center, Department of Psychiatry, Pennsylvania State University, Milton S. Hershey Medical Center, Hershey, Pennsylvania 17033

Robert D. Lindeman, Oklahoma City Veterans Administration Hospital, and, Departments of Medicine and Physiology, University of Oklahoma Health Sciences Center, Oklahoma City, Oklahoma 73104

Bernard S. Linn, Department of Surgery, University of Miami School of Medicine, and, Veterans Administration Hospital, Miami, Florida 33152

David P. Richey, Smith, Kline & French Laboratories, Philadelphia, Pennsylvania 19101

Morris Rockstein, Department of Physiology and Biophysics, University of Miami School of Medicine, Miami, Florida 33152

Ruth B. Weg, Department of Biology, Andrus Gerontology Center, University of Southern California, Los Angeles, California 90007

PREFACE

As in past years, this, the fifth publication in a series of proceedings of annual symposia, represents the discussions of a gathering of scientists, in this case chiefly clinical research gerontologists, all of whom have made recognized contributions to their respective fields of biomedical gerontology. What we believe to be especially unique about the presentations by these participants is their basic approach to major functional changes with age in humans, from the standpoint of gross and microanatomical (even ultrastructural) changes, their biochemical concomitants, aside from the actual known functional decrements for each of the major areas being discussed. Thus, although primarily concerned with a particular major human system or clinical area of gerontology, the inclusion, in most instances, of the underlying cellular bases for the age-related decrements of such major biological functions, discussed by each of the participants, reflects the basic theme of cellular aging which this Training Program has as its research training objective.

As in the case of past symposia of this series, each of the several areas of human aging covered at this meeting is discussed by an individual who is both clinically as well as scientifically competent to do so. The reader will note, moreover, that a number of misconceptions concerning aging, for such phenomena as atherosclerosis, kidney function, the effects of drugs, sleep, sexuality, osteoporosis, cardiac function, and surgery, in the elderly, are laid to rest by the incisive and highly critical treatment of the several experts participating in this important symposium.

In making available these proceedings in published form, the Editors hope that the contents of this volume will serve to attract not only more basic scientists but clinical researchers, particularly to work in this challenging research field of biomedical gerontology.

Ralph Goldman
Morris Rockstein

ACKNOWLEDGMENTS

The Editors owe special thanks to Mrs. Estella Cooney for her dedication to producing, as in the past, the final published version of these proceedings in both editing and typing of the camera copy for this publication. We are particularly grateful to Marvin L. Sussman, our Associate Editor, for his tireless and dedicated efforts in the joint editing of these proceedings from their initial manuscript form to the final camera copy of this published work.

The Training Program is deeply appreciative of the generosity of the American Committee for the Weizmann Institute of Science in making possible the participation of Dr. David Danon in this Symposium. It must also express its gratitude to Dr. Alfred T. Sapse, President of Rom-Amer Pharmaceuticals Ltd., Beverly Hills, California, and to the staff of Academic Press, whose generous contributions helped make this a successful conference, as well as the publication of these proceedings possible.

The Symposium from which this publication resulted was supported, for the most part, by funds from the National Institute of Child Health and Human Development (Training Program in Cellular Aging) Grant No. HD 00142, also in part by the University of Miami Center for Urban and Regional Studies Aging Programs, and, by the University of Miami Department of Physiology and Biophysics, Professor Werner R. Loewenstein, Chairman.

THE BIOLOGY OF AGING IN HUMANS - AN OVERVIEW

Morris Rockstein

Department of Physiology and Biophysics
University of Miami School of Medicine
Miami, Florida

  In his continued search for extending his longevity as well as retarding if not preventing the aging process <u>per se</u>, only during the past two and a half decades has modern man been truly sufficiently concerned to encourage as well as undertake research in the nature of the aging process. Perforce much of our emphasis has had to be directed to research in lower animals, particularly as regards homologous (or at least analogous) systems, organs and cells. In humans, characterization of the gradual and often subtle changes in the structure of organ systems with age, with a resulting functional deterioration, has been possible primarily through limited longitudinal studies (following the same person throughout his entire life, hopefully beginning, at the very least, with middle age). On the other hand, cross-sectional studies (obtaining data from many individuals for specific age groups in a given population - the customary approach to aging research in lower animals), certainly, have had to be the primary basis for accumulating such data in humans.
  In the United States today, with over 20 million men and women age 65 and over and 15 million plus age 75 and over, it is obvious that there is a need for a complete understanding of the facts of "normal" aging, and, to an even greater extent, of the pathology of human aging. As a result of the elimination of many childhood diseases as well as the general improvement of basic medical care, the mean longevity of man has increased over the past 50 years. Consequently, the general practitioner or the geriatrician is confronted daily with increasingly larger numbers of cases involving persons 65 years of age and above, particularly in such states as Florida, Nebraska, Iowa, and Arkansas, where the percentage of such older individuals is greatest (in descending order) as well as in New York, California, Illinois, Ohio, and Texas, the states with the largest <u>absolute</u> numbers of individuals 65 years of age or over. From the standpoint of the national

economy, it is interesting to note that persons under 65 spent as little as $226 per capita per year on medical care; on the other hand, men and women 65 years of age and over spent $791 per person per year in 1970, the great majority of which came from Medicare and Medicaid. Thus, public programs combined to pay 2/3 of the bill for the health care costs of the elderly.

Some years ago, I was asked to present a summary of the known facts of human aging before a lay group in connection with the twentieth Annual Meeting of the Gerontological Society held in St. Petersburg, Florida in 1967 (Rockstein, 1968). In the 8 years since that conference, some limited progress has been added to our understanding of the facts of aging in humans. However, although the highly competent authorities speaking at this two-day symposium will elaborate upon the various aspects of aging in humans, I am exercising my prerogative as Chairman to introduce this two-day meeting by this concise summary of the more general known facts of human aging.

It is true that some people think of aging in terms of such obvious changes as farsightedness or presbyopia, loss of hearing, graying of the hair and wrinkling of the skin. Others frequently speak of diseases of old age, but there are, at best, only diseases as many (and chiefly of the same kind) as those occurring in middle age, if not earlier.

On the other hand, there are indeed a considerable number of structural and functional changes in the human body, some occurring earlier, others later, in different human beings, which we all agree can be truly labeled aging or senescence (see Korenchevsky, 1961; Anon., 1966).

How then does an older person differ from a young or mature individual?

1. Outward appearance - The outer appearance of an individual, unless altered by "cosmetic surgical procedure", can be a good index of the rate of aging of that particular individual. The skin becomes wrinkled, is generally less elastic and dry, with localized pigment plaques particularly typical of advanced age. The small blood vessels of the skin become increasingly fragile so that small bruises produce black and blue spots (ecchymoses) more readily than in younger individuals. The hair becomes gray to white and usually thinner in distribution in women as well as men. Sweating is also considerably reduced in older persons. Finally, an older person, primarily due to the weakening of certain muscles, tends to be bent over and stooped in appearance.

2. The muscles - A common manifestation of senescence is a decrease in muscular strength, endurance and, certainly, agility, aside from slower reaction time. The last-mentioned is in part due to changes in the nervous system, to be discussed below. Structurally, this wasting of muscle is reflected in the decreased number of muscle fibers due to the inability of muscle to regenerate, with fibrous tissues secondarily replacing the contractile elements. Accordingly, the hands become thinner and bonier, with the arm and leg muscles becoming reduced in size and flabby in appearance.

3. Skeletal system - As it has been earlier indicated, the posture tends to become one of stooping, with the head and neck held somewhat forward and the upper limbs bent. This is due in part to not only muscle shrinkage, but also the decrease in elasticity and calcification of ligaments, shrinkage and sclerosis of tendons, as well as changes in the vertebral column, including flattening of the intervertebral discs. The average height of aging individuals, accordingly, diminishes somewhat with advancing age. Although senile osteoporosis (to be discussed later in greater detail by Dr. Garn) was once considered an inevitable consequence of getting older, the increased number of observations on the (ever increasing number of) older individuals has led to the understanding of this particular condition as a disease rather than as a normal "aging phenomenon". In general, however, there is evidence of a fairly universally distributed increasing negative calcium balance with advancing age which Garn prefers to call "adult bone-loss", amelioration of which, by calcium supplementation, is questionable (see Garn's chapter).

4. Nervous system - It is generally acknowledged there is a loss in the total number of brain cells and their fibers with advancing age, aside from the more dramatic effects of hardening of the vessels of the brain in very advanced age. Thus, all humans, like lower animals, show a decline in total number of brain cells with age, sometimes in specific areas of the brain only (Brody, 1973), with a loss of brain weight of about 20 to 25% from maturity to age 90 or over. In general, there is a gradual failing of memory capacity with advancing age, particularly in short-term memory later in life, upon which Dr. Goldfarb will elaborate in his chapter.

Physiologically, conduction velocity has been reported to decrease in individuals with advancing age. In this connection, voluntary motor movements have been observed to slow down and reaction time to be reduced for such movements with an increase in reflex time for reflex skeletal muscle responses in older persons (see Rockstein and Sussman, 1973).

5. Special senses - As far as responsiveness to the external environment is concerned, the sense of touch begins to be somewhat dulled after 50, the feet losing their sensitivity to touch and vibration faster than the hands. Concomitantly, pain thresholds actually rise in individuals over 50, which, of course, increases the likelihood of ignoring any kind of pathological state in which pain may be an important signal. This may result in the delay of treatment and, therefore, aggravation of such pathological conditions.

Presbyopia or farsightedness is probably the most universally distributed manifestation of aging occurring between 40 and 50 years of age, with cataracts occurring in 33% of elderly persons. At the same time, adaptation to the dark as well as acuity of night vision show a gradual failing with advancing age.

As in the case of generalized neuronal loss with advancing age, loss of hearing may be a slow, but progressive manifestation of the aging process, particularly as regards the high frequency tones first.

Likewise, there is a progressive loss in the aging person's capacity for taste as well as smell. In this connection, there is concrete evidence for a loss in a number of taste buds per papilla from 30 to 75 years of age by approximately one-third, whereas the number of fibers in the olfactory nerve diminishes steadily as we get older, as well. This combined reduction in sensitivity of senses concerned with food intake must compound the problems of the dietary needs of the older individual, particularly those who are living alone.

Balance disturbances, probably responsible for the high rate of accidents among the elderly, is likewise a physiological accompaniment of advancing age. This is most probably due to degenerative changes in the neuronal elements of the inner ear.

The general slowing down of skeletal muscle responses, discussed earlier, is also due in part to both sensory-perception losses, on the one hand, as well as to diminished number of central nervous system neurones as well.

6. Cardiovascular system - As Dr. Harris will recount in greater detail, the effectiveness of the heart as a pump is markedly reduced in later years, despite the fact that there is only a modest loss in the total cardiac muscle mass with age. It is particularly manifest in the drastic reduction in the cardiac output of the heart, at rest, past 65 years of age. This may indeed be due chiefly to the progressive age-related increase in resistance of the arterial

vessels to blood flow. In the last-mentioned connection, the normal adult male, with a blood pressure of 120/75 at age 25, will show a blood pressure reading of approximately 160/90 after age 65. Moreover, postural hypotension, the sudden drop in blood pressure which occurs when an individual rises suddenly from a reclining position, is much more severe in individuals over 65 years of age, chiefly attributable to aging of the nervous system concerned with reflex control of blood pressure.

7. Respiratory system - Another well-documented manifestation of aging in all humans is the sum total of changes in structure and function of the lungs. Thus, both the total capacity as well as the vital capacity of the lungs decrease with age. This is due in part to the fact that there is weakening in the muscles which are used in lifting the rib cage, increasing obesity, and sometimes skeletal abnormalities of the rib cage developing as a person grows older. There is likewise a reduction in the total number of alveoli, as well as reduction in flexibility or expandability of the lungs, in turn due to changes in the elastic fibers of the bronchioles, as well as weakening of the external intercostal muscles. There is also an increase in thickening of the membranes lining the air sacs of the lungs, so that the rate of movement of gases across these membranes into the vascular supply of the alveoli is reduced considerably. Emphysema is particularly common in older people, but at an earlier age and in an ultimately more severe form in heavy smokers.

8. Digestion - Aside from the contribution of poor teeth or ill-fitting dentures, as well as poor diets for a number of reasons, digestive difficulties and intestinal upsets are a major problem of the elderly, due in part to reduced motility of the stomach and a reduction in the peristaltic activity of the intestine and colon. Constipation, a common digestive, alimentary tract dysfunction in older persons, results from the above as well as from a modified diet.

9. Urinary tract - As Dr. Richey will discuss in greater detail, the rate of filtering by the kidney in persons over 80 is reduced by about 50% of the rate at 25 years of age. This observed change in filtration rate is a reflection of an identical reduction in the actual blood flow through the kidneys over this span of years. Excessive urination and night time micturition are common among the aged, but particularly in male humans over 55 years of age where prostatic

enlargement (occurring in about 76% of the male population over 55 years of age) is the cause of such polyuria.

10. Reproductive organs - As Dr. Weg will indicate, the climacteric, occurring in the late 40s and early 50s in the human female, is less demonstrable and occurs at a much later age in the human male. At the same time, the extent of atrophy of the male reproductive organs following menopause is considerably less than that observed in the postmenopausal woman.

11. Endocrines - Aside from the age-related changes in sexual hormones associated with the aging of the reproductive system, both the thyroid stimulating hormone of the pituitary and the thyroid hormone secreted by the thyroid glands themselves, show a decline with advancing age. This is functionally reflected in the steady decrease in the basal metabolic rate, from age 30 to age 70 by as much as 20%.

Probably the most generalized physiological manifestation of aging is the relative inability to adapt to or respond to stress to the same extent as in one's younger years. This is particularly true for such phenomena as temperature regulation, displacement of the blood pH, the rate of return to equilibrium of which is much slower in older people than in young.

It is a well known fact that aging humans show an increasing tendency to chilling with advancing age. This is manifest in the inability to maintain a constant body temperature, particularly when the external, ambient temperature falls below 65° F. This is doubtless due, in part, to the falling basal metabolic rate as well as the failing effectiveness of the nervous system involved. Indeed, rectal temperatures in very old persons may fall to temperatures well below 90° F. This is due in part to the lowered rate of metabolism as well as the likelihood of improper nutrition in such individuals.

The response to intravenous administration of glucose (the glucose tolerance test) shows marked reduction in older individuals. Shock and Andres (1968) explained this on the basis of a reduction in the sensitivity of the beta cells of the pancreas to blood sugar levels with advancing age.

In closing, may I emphasize a point made by this author that all organs do not age at the same rate in one individual nor does a particular organ system age at the same rate in different individuals. This observation calls to mind the commentary by the late Otto Loewi, a cherished colleague, while I served on the faculty at the New York University School of Medicine, relating his concerns about growing old, as he passed his 80th birthday. To Dr. Loewi there were three stages of growing old, "The first," he said, "is that time when one has indeed aged but when he alone is aware of the fact that he has grown old, the second is when an individual realizes that he has grown old and the rest of the world is also aware of this, and, finally, the third stage of senescence is that time when the individual who has grown old is no longer aware of the fact that he is old, but the rest of the world is patently aware of it"!

REFERENCES

Anon. (1966). "Working with Older People: A Guide to Practice", Vol. I, "The Practitioner and the Elderly", U. S. Department HEW, Washington, D. C.

Brody, H. (1973). In "Development and Aging in the Nervous System" (M. Rockstein, and M. L. Sussman, eds.), pp. 121-133, Academic Press, New York.

Korenchevsky, V. (1961). "Physiological and Pathological Ageing" (G. H. Bourne, ed.), S. Karger, Basel, Switzerland.

Rockstein, M. (1968). The Gerontologist 8, 124.

Rockstein, M., and Sussman, M. L. (eds.) (1973). "Development and Aging in the Nervous System". Academic Press, New York.

Shock, N. W., and Andres, R. (1968). In "Adaptive Capacities of an Aging Organism" (D. F. Chebotarev, ed.), pp. 235-254, Acad. Sci., USSR, Kiev.

CHRONOLOGIC VS. BIOLOGIC AGE
IN GERIATRIC PATIENTS*

Bernard S. Linn, M.D.

Department of Surgery
University of Miami School of Medicine
and
Veterans Administration Hospital
Miami, Florida

Clinicians are called upon every day to make decisions about the management of their patients. Usually, the first bit of information in the patient's workup is his or her age, i.e. "37-year-old black male with chief complaint of cough, 3 mos..."; "56-year-old white female with chief complaint of abdominal pain, 6 hours...". Unfortunately, although a patient's chronologic age may be the simplest index of aging known, it may not always be the most useful criterion. Some persons are evidently "old" at 50, while others are surprisingly "young" at 80. The index of aging being estimated here by the patient's overall appearance is not chronologic age, but rather the physiologic or so-called "biologic" age of the individual patient. For purposes of this paper, I would like to focus upon three specific areas:

1. the influence of age, in and of itself, on physiology and outcome of disease,

2. some ways in which biologic age have been measured and used clinically to date, and

3. an overview which fits biologic age into the perspective of survival, longevity, and aging.

Influence of Age on Physiology and Outcome of Disease

The classical studies of Shock (1962) described the occurrence of many organ systems manifesting age-related

---

* Work supported in part by VA 8200 Research and Development funds.

declines in function and homeostatic mechanisms that usually begin shortly after maturity and progress into old age. In comparing organ functions between ages from 30 to 90, he noted an almost linear deterioration of function for various organ systems, even though their rates of deterioration did vary. For example, the cardiac index fell 30%, vital breathing capacity dropped over 50%, and renal plasma flow (which is dependent, however, on the technique employed in its measurement) declined 50 to 60%. The proportion of these declines were caused by what might be termed "normal physiologic aging" as compared to pathologic-specific disease processes, although of great interest from a gerontologic point of view, is not really so much a relevant clinical issue since regardless of whether the change is physiologic or pathologic, any decrease in function with time means an increase in biologic age.

There are, however, two much more relevant clinical questions one might ask. The first is whether these changes, that can inevitably be observed in association with increasing age, are really normal and physiologic for that given particular age group, or whether they are abnormal and pathologic. An excellent example of this common and somewhat semantic problem which confronts the clinician, who is trying to decide whether disease is or is not present, has been given by Andres (1967). Andres pointed out that if one applies the usual "normal" glucose tolerance values to a geriatric population, that 50% of this group would have to be classified as latent biochemical diabetics, when, in point of fact, the actual prevalence of frank diabetes in this same age group is only 8%. On the other hand, if one were to define "normal" by the usual technique of computing the group mean and identifying abnormals as greater than two standard deviations from this mean, only 2.3% of this group (less than a third of the prevalence) would be identified as having latent diabetes. Some additional judgment is therefore still required as to where the true dividing line is between the physiologic and pathologic changes of the aging process, although this type of approach does define the two extremes of "normal" very nicely.

The second relevant clinical question which one might ask in relation to the functional declines associated with increasing chronologic age is whether these declines occur continuously or in sporadic bursts, or in some combination of the two. In this regard, Lapides and Zierdt (1967) pointed out that a high proporation (a third) of their elderly urologic patients had "normal" clinical renal functions. They therefore questioned whether the observed changes might

not, in greatest measure, be on an individual basis because
of periodic occurrence of disease rather than being a more
continuous process with occasional incremental increases due
to disease. Put another way, they were asking whether the
decline in function related to age groups simply reflected
a decreasing proportion of normal patients in the older
groups as increasing number of members among the group
develop impairments due to actual episodes of disease. Although this question cannot be answered precisely without
additional specific longitudinal studies, certainly one's
clinical "hunch" is that there must be some element of continuous decline, since a man of 80, regardless of how unremarkable his total past medical history may be, will never
be confused with a man of 30, regardless of how remarkably
complicated the younger man's lifelong disease processes may
have been. In point of fact, some clinicians do give
evidence, by the increasing therapeutic vigor they use with
some of their older patients, of their confidence in the
residual stamina of many of their elderly patients.

A good example of this decreasing influence of age in
making clinical decisions in relation to surgery has been
crystallized clearly in the following excerpt from Ochsner
(1967):

> "In 1927, as a young professor of surgery at the
> Tulane Medical School, I taught and practiced
> that an elective operation for inguinal hernia
> in a patient older than 50 years of age was not
> justified... Today age is in no way a surgical
> contraindication."

The chief justification for this kind of attitude is, of
course, the increasingly lower rates of operative morbidity
and mortality being reported in relation to surgery in the
aged. Surgical outcomes are also being reported specifically
for octagenerians, nonagenerians, and even centenarians. In
spite of this, one can also find evidence, some of which will
be mentioned later, that many clinicians still favor chronologic age per se as an indication (even if unspoken) against
more vigorous management.

Improved clinical results alone are all well and good,
but such improvement could just as well be a testimony to
advances in medical techniques as to the stamina of the
elderly. Thus, it is important to look for other data concerning the relationship of age to outcome of surgery that
would be less ambiguous, and perhaps also somewhat more
germaine to basic gerontology. Along these lines, there is

a growing body of evidence, when one compares outcomes in geriatric versus younger patients, with even limited controls for degree of severity of illness, that results are frequently not very different. For example, in 292 consecutive cardiac arrests, age was not found to discriminate between those patients who were successfully resuscitated and those who were not (Linn and Yurt, 1970). Relative five-year survival rates from internal cancers were found to be similar for most age groups when compared on the basis of comparable clinical stages of the disease (Anonymous, 1969). Even though the gross mortality rate in a series of 272 operations for peptic ulcer was greater among older patients, there were no significant differences in outcome related to age in the non-emergency surgery group (Linn, 1975). The fact that older patients had a greater percentage of operations done as emergencies (and emergencies invariably have two to four times greater mortality than comparable elective surgery) raises the possibility of some reluctance among clinicians to operate as readily on their older as on their younger patients. However, without also weighing the severity of concomitant illnesses, this cannot be stated with certainty.

The final evidence to be cited in relation to the question of how chronologic age influences disease outcome relates to burns in the elderly (Linn, 1974). The traditional dictum about outcome in burns states that two variables, age and percent of body surface area affected, are the major predictors of survival or non-survival. In this review of 1600 burn admissions over a one-year period in Florida, if one corrected for percent body surface area burned, there was a marked reduction in the influence of age on outcome. In this study, there was also considerable circumstantial evidence that age may still have influenced clinicians to use less aggressive management in the older patients, in that significantly poorer medical records and significantly less essential debridement and grafting were found among the older patients for comparable burn involvements. In summary then, both clinical practice as well as clinical investigations have provided considerable evidence that chronologic age alone, independent of past medical history and severity of illness, has much less influence than expected originally on disease outcome.

Measurement of Biologic Age

Rockstein (1968) has concisely reviewed some of the correlates of biologic aging, including such widely divergent individual variables as skin changes, graying of hair, musculoskeletal atrophy, sensory and reflex decrements, loss of teeth, cardiovascular and respiratory changes, reduced peristalsis, menopause, and memory loss. A major problem still remaining for the clinician is one of categorizing these variables in some way as to provide a more useful index to the overall level of aging which has occurred in a given individual.

In reviewing the specific instruments developed to date, which might serve as such an index of biologic aging, one is struck by the relative paucity of devices that exist for rating physical, as opposed to psychological pathology. Perhaps this is all the more surprising in light of the fact that physical measures deal with a far more concrete and verifiable area. At any rate, an early attempt and perhaps still the most widely used instrument in this sphere is the Cornell Medical Index (Brodman et al., 1955) in which the total score itself is indicative of symptomatic physical status and is derived from the patient's self-report in the answers to 195 questions dealing with the presence or absence of particular symptoms. The most evident immediate problems precluding the generalized use of this test are its length and lack of validation as an index associated with biologic age and ultimate mortality. Another instrument, reported by Hollingsworth et al. (1965), is a product of their work with the Atomic Bomb Casualty Commission in Japan, and defines nine concomitant tests (ranging from measurement of skin elasticity, systolic blood pressure through grip strength, vibration sense, and serum cholesterol levels) to provide feasible serial data for statistical formulation of biologic age. Even ignoring the pragmatic problem that some of these measurements (such as grip strength, vital capacity, light perception time, and audiometry) are not usually part of routine physical exams, the authors themselves note that the all-important validation of these tests by correlation with ultimate mortality was likewise still to be done.

Another approach to measurement of biologic age derives from the hypothesis of Jones (1959) in which the force of mortality is regarded as the progressive development of various kinds of impairments and that the death rate is therefore a measure of the cumulative effects of each such incremental impairment which occurs in an individual's lifetime. Our own interest in biologic age, which began in 1964, led to the development of a Cumulative Illness Rating Scale (CIRS) (Linn et al., 1968) which was designed as a simple way in which the clinician could quantify impairment. There is some importance in distinguishing between the more numerous measures of disability, which refer to adequacy of performance in areas of functions (such as eating, dressing, or

toileting) which can be rated by anyone familiar with the
patient, and measures of impairment which call for the
clinician's estimate of the degree of underlying pathophysiology based on his knowledge of the patient's symptoms, signs,
and laboratory findings. Not surprisingly, the ability of
impairment ratings to predict mortality has been found to
exceed that of disability ratings (Linn et al., 1971). This
is not stated to condemn disability ratings, which have certainly been quite useful for many purposes, but to stress
that the quantification-of-impairment has been almost totally
neglected as evidenced by the dearth of impairment rating
scales. The CIRS drew upon the observations that practicing
clinicians are involved daily in decisions relating to diagnosis and prognosis which imply quantitative estimates of
organ function and cumulative impairment. In the present
version of the scale, there are 13 items grouped by body
systems, with vital organs rated separately. The doctor rates
each item on a 5-point degree of severity scale, ranging from
0 (none) to 4 (extremely severe). The primary function of the
scale is to serve as a brief assessment tool applicable to the
study of biologic aging. After first establishing reliability
and validity, the CIRS was used to test the hypothesis that
persons who lived to extremely old age were biologically more
elite (Linn et al., 1967) in that they had no more cumulative
impairment than "younger" older subjects. It was found that
although specific kinds of illness were related to each of
three different age groups of living subjects (75 and over,
65-74, and 55-64) there were no significant differences between groups in total CIRS scores. A second study was done
along these lines (Linn et al., 1969) using mortality as an
outcome criteria to test the relationship of degree of cumulatime pathology to death in these same three age groups.
Similar findings occurred with different pathology patterns
related to age groups but with no significant differences in
total CIRS scores (although they were significantly higher
than the first study). One conclusion, not meant to be
facetious, was that when individuals reached a certain score
for cumulative pathology, their "number was up"--literally.
Individuals in the older age group had significantly more
cases of pulmonary embolism, hernia, and carcinoma of the
prostate. The middle group had significantly more myocardial
infarctions and diabetes, while alcoholism, cirrhosis and
injuries occurred most frequently in the younger patients.
The recurrent finding in both studies of no variation between
groups in relation to degree of accumulated pathology led to
a third study to test the hypothesis that the actual timing
of illnesses differed between older and younger subjects who
died (Linn et al., 1972). In the older subjects, illnesses

were found to cluster around the closing years of life, whereas in younger subjects the onset was significantly earlier and the dispersion significantly greater. It was concluded that the older patients were a biologically elite group who were largely free from the usual "killer" diseases and who suffered more from a terminal chain of degenerative type diseases. In contrast, their younger counterparts in the study had a greater spread of illness throughout their lifetime with one of the more acute "killer" diseases occurring near the time of their death.

Fitting Biologic Age into the Perspective of Survival and Aging

Even though the CIRS has been of considerable help in pointing to some of the biologic differences and similarities between groups with different chronologic ages, there is still a great deal it doesn't do. For one thing, the old still had obvious differences in appearance from the young which the CIRS did not measure. Of even greater importance perhaps was the fact that there were individual extremes in the variance of CIRS scores within each group that raised questions about why these patients, as individuals, behaved differently from what one might expect from their scores. One very good reason for this variation is that any measure of cumulative pathology alone, however great its accuracy may ultimately be refined, is not a sufficiently comprehensive measure of biologic age to predict survival fully. This point will now be developed further in this section of the paper.

Let us take the simplest possible overview and presume that each individual is born with a certain threshold of resistance to the potential impairments of aging and illness in the lifetime ahead. With each increase in cumulative pathology throughout each person's lifetime, there is a concomitant decrease in residual adaptability to additional new impairments. Death occurs at the point when severity of a new impairment exceeds the individual's threshold of resistance.

Figure 1 diagrams these basic phenomena and interrelationships of aging which affect each individual. In this figure, the vertical scale provides a measure either of the amount of resistance to impairment or of the amount of impairment itself. Increasing chronologic age (or time) is plotted along the horizontal axis. The diagonal line (or incremental steps) which depict the rate of impairment accumulation can in one sense be thought of as the force of mortality for that individual patient. Notice that death occurs at the point where cumulative impairment exceeds the threshold of resistance. Hence death occurs when stress produces sufficient cumulative impairment (under the rate of impairment line) to use up all of the residual adaptability (over the rate of impairment line). Longer life will result in individuals with greater thresholds of resistance and/or lower rates of impairment, and conversely, shorter life will result when the opposite occurs. Viewed in this perspective, an individual's biologic age could be obtained which would provide a more accurate index of total aging processes if it takes account not only of cumulative pathology but of residual adaptability as well

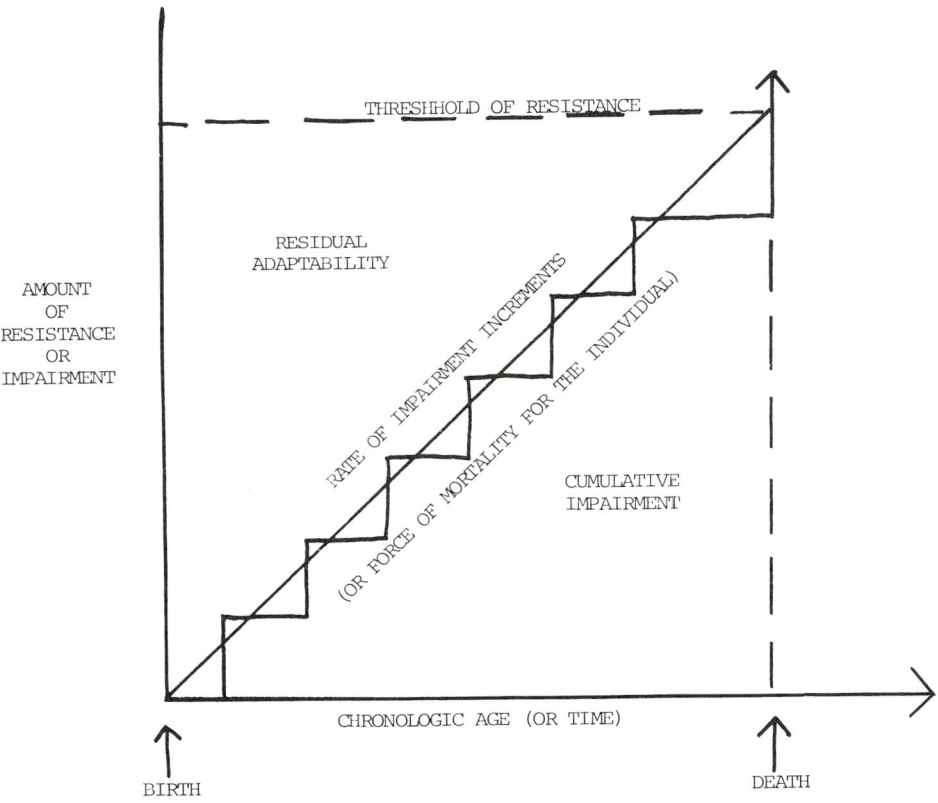

Fig. 1 A scheme for the lifetime of an individual which depicts: A) total residual adaptability (present at birth) being gradually used up as total impairment accumulates over the years; B) death occurring at the point when there is no more residual adaptability, i.e., when cumulative impairment exceeds threshold of resistance.

Obviously, the most important tool the clinician could extract from this conceptualization of the aging process is some index of biologic age that would be of help in decisions relative to management and prognosis. Qualitatively, nothing has been said that is at all very strange to the clinician. For what has been called "cumulative past impairment", he calls "past medical history". "New impairment" is what he calls "present illness", and the clinician may view "residual adaptability" as just that or perhaps as "present condition", so that the physician's prognosis is simply a composite of the severity of past and present illnesses coupled with his judgment of the patient's present condition.

To assist physicians in their practice as well as to provide a means for better comparing groups of individuals in terms of their biologic age, it would be helpful if some scale for measuring biologic age could ultimately be developed. Actually, this may not be so far in the future. Cumulative past and present impairment can be measured to some extent by instruments such as the CIRS. In addition, the recent emphasis in evaluation of medical care and interest in trauma management has resulted in reports of two new indexes for severity of trauma in just the past year (Cowley et al., 1974; Baker et al., 1974). Although both of these scales were specifically developed to measure the severity of injury, they are, in fact, also measuring or at least correlating directly with the severity of impairment produced by the injury. By looking again at figure 1, one can see that what is needed still in order to project any individual's survival once past and present impairments are known, would be some measure for that same individual of either their threshold of resistance or of their residual adaptability. Although one could possibly think in terms of an individual's threshold of resistance as a correlate of information related to the health histories of their parents, grandparents, and siblings, the residual adaptability might be more useful as a clinical tool, particularly if measured in terms of vital organ function and reserve. In either case, adding a measure for threshold of resistance or for residual adaptability would, if coupled to what is already measurable about impairment, seem to offer a far more precise index of an individual's biologic age in the perspective of their overall longevity prospects.

REFERENCES

Andres, R. (1967). *Mayo Clin. Proc.* 42, 674.
Anonymous (1969). *Gerifacts* August, p. 204.
Baker, S. P., O'Neill, B., Haddon, W., and Long, W. B. (1974). *J. Trauma* 14, 187.
Brodman, L., Erdman, A. J., and Wolff, H. G. (1955). In "Cornell Medical Index Manual", Cornell University Press, New York.
Cowley, R. A., Sacco, W. J., Gill, W., Champion, H. R., Long, W. B., Copes, W. S., Goldfarb, M. A., and Sperrazza, J. (1974). *J. Trauma* 14, 1029.
Hollingsworth, J. W., Hashizume, A., and Jablon, S. (1965). *Yale J. Biol. Med.* 38, 11.
Jones, H. B. (1959). In "Handbook of Aging" (J. Birren, ed.), pp. 336-363, University of Chicago Press, Chicago.
Lapides, J., and Zierdt, D. (1967). *J. Am. Med. Assoc.* 201, 152.
Linn, B. S. (1974). *Gerontologist* 14, 37.
Linn, B. S. (1975). To be presented at the 10th International Congress of Gerontology, June 22, 1975, Jerusalem, Israel.
Linn, B. S., and Yurt, R. W. (1970). *Brit. Med. J.* 2, 25.
Linn, B. S., Linn, M. W., and Gurel, L. (1968). *J. Am. Geriat. Soc.* 16, 622.
Linn, B. S., Linn, M. W., and Gurel, L. (1969). *Gerontol. Clin.* 11, 362.
Linn, B. S., Linn, M. W., and Gurel, L. (1971). In "Prediction of Life Span" (E. Palmore and F. Jeffers, eds.), pp. 51-59, D. C. Heath Company, Lexington, Massachusetts.
Linn, M. W., Linn, B. S., and Gurel, L. (1967). *Geriatrics* 22, 134.
Linn, M. W., Linn, B. S., and Gurel, L. (1972). *Geriatrics* 27, 67.
Ochsner, A. (1967). *Geriatrics* 22, 121.
Rockstein, M. (1968). *Gerontologist* 8, 124.
Shock, N. W. (1962). In "Biology of Aging" (B. L. Strehler, ed.), p. 22, American Institute of Biological Sciences, Washington, D. C.

AGE CHANGES IN RENAL FUNCTION

Robert D. Lindeman, M. D.*

Medical Service, Oklahoma City Veterans
Administration Hospital and
Departments of Medicine and Physiology,
University of Oklahoma Health Sciences Center,
Oklahoma City, Oklahoma 73104

The kidney is responsible for elimination from the body of most of the non-volatile waste products of metabolism. Equally important is its role in maintenance of a constant internal environment of fluid volume and electrolyte and hydrogen ion concentrations. By formation of large volumes of an ultrafiltrate of plasma in the glomerular capillary beds followed by selective reabsorption and secretion of electrolytes and other ions in the tubule, the normal kidney possesses an enormous capacity to maintain precisely fluid, electrolyte and acid-base balance. Most imbalances result not from loss of renal function or reserve, but rather from extrarenal pathology that initiates transmission of inappropriate or faulty information to renal regulatory mechanisms.

The blood vessels, glomeruli, tubules and interstitium are potential sites of primary involvement in different renal diseases. Regardless of the anatomic structure primarily affected, most chronic conditions ultimately evolve with destruction of entire nephrons. In a number of cross-sectional studies plotting different aspects of renal function against age, there has been demonstrated a progressive decrease with age after the age of 40 years. The decreases with age in all parameters studied have paralleled the decreases in renal plasma flow and glomerular filtration rate. Whether the observed decrease in renal function associated with age is the result of intercurrent pathologic processes such as ischemia due to obliteration of vascular blood supply or infection in the renal parenchyma or is the

---

*Professor of Medicine and Physiology; Chief, Nephrology Section, University of Oklahoma College of Medicine; Associate Chief of Staff, Oklahoma City Veterans Administration Hospital.

result of some more physiologic involutional process remains undetermined.

Normally, despite a decrease in renal function with age, the integrity of the volume and composition of the body fluids is maintained under basal conditions. However, when disease or environmental stress results in a greater demand on renal function, renal adjustments are slower in older persons than they are in the young, healthy individual.

Specific Renal Functional Changes with Age

Six separate measures of renal function have been selected for discussion in this review, as shown in Table I.

Table I

Measures of Renal Function

1. Glomerular Filtration Rate
2. Renal Plasma and Blood Flow
3. Maximum Tubular Transport Capacity
4. Concentrating and Diluting Ability
5. Ability to Acidify Urine
6. Glomerular Permeability

1. <u>Glomerular Filtration Rate</u>. The most frequently utilized and most useful measure of renal function is an estimate of the glomerular filtration rate (GFR). The rate at which glomerular filtrate is formed is dependent primarily upon the rate of blood flow through the kidney, normally about 20% of the plasma circulating through the kidney. The inulin clearance has been used in most research studies to measure glomerular filtration rate and all indications are that it is freely filtered and neither reabsorbed nor secreted and therefore is an accurate measure of glomerular filtration rate. Several isotopes such as I^{131} or I^{125} iothalamate have been used more recently with comparable accuracy and precision. The urinary clearances of endogenous

metabolic waste products such as urea and creatinine approximate those of inulin and are much easier to obtain in studies where accuracy and precision are not as critical.

Davies and Shock (1950) reported that a decrease in inulin clearance occurred with age in 70 male subjects, age 20 to 90 years, who had no history or clinical evidence of renal or cardiovascular disease, hypertension or acute illness. Incorporating these findings along with data reported on normal male subjects in 36 additional studies where age was recorded with individual inulin clearances, Wesson (1969) found an accelerating decrease in renal function with increasing age (figure 1).

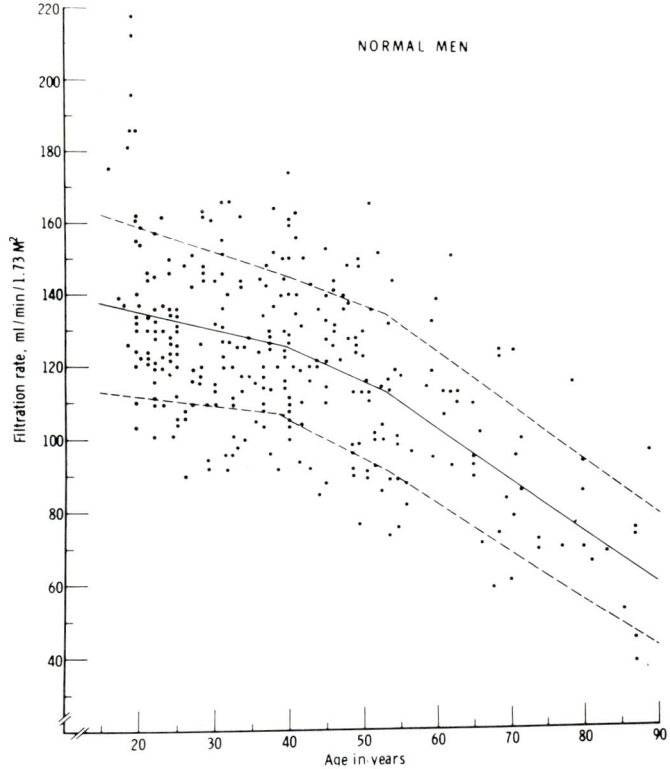

Fig. 1 Glomerular filtration rates (inulin clearances) per 1.73 M^2 in normal men vs. age in 38 studies reported by Wesson (1969). The solid and broken lines represent mean $\pm$ one standard deviation.

These observations have been further confirmed in studies underway at the Gerontology Research Institute in Baltimore (Shock, 1967) where over 500 male subjects have had serial endogenous creatinine clearances repeated at 18 month intervals over a 15 year period.

    2. <u>Renal Plasma and Blood Flow</u>. The amount of plasma or blood perfusing the kidney can be estimated by measuring para-aminohippuric acid (PAH) or diodrast clearance. Davies and Shock (1950), confirming the work of Bradley (1947), showed the extraction ratio for PAH at low arterial PAH concentrations was approximately 92% in 27 subjects of varying age and this extraction ratio was not affected by age. This means that 92% of the PAH entering the kidney on the arterial side was removed in one passage through the kidney or that 8% of the arterial concentration was found in the venous side. The mean decrease in renal plasma flow with age as measured by PAH clearance was slightly greater than was the decrease in inulin clearance with age (Davies and Shock, 1950; Wesson, 1969).

    The decrease in renal blood flow with age without a decrease in blood pressure suggests either vascular obliteration due to intraluminal pathology (sclerosis, atheromata, clot, etc.) or an increase in renal vascular resistance. Since renal blood flow can be transiently increased by administration of pyrogen in both young and old subjects (McDonald <u>et al</u>., 1951), a reversible or vasoconstrictive component may be important in the regulation of the renal circulation in both age groups. Actually, administration of pyrogen produces a greater vasodilatation in the afferent arterioles of the kidney in the older than the younger person suggesting a greater vasoconstriction exists in the resting state in the older subjects. The reason for this increased afferent vasoconstriction in the elderly remains unclear. One might speculate that cardiac output also decreases with age making it necessary to vasoconstrict renal arterioles in order to better maintain the blood supply to other vital organs.

    Hollenberg <u>et al</u>. (1974) felt their findings of an increasing filtration fraction with age coupled with their xenon washout data indicated that the perfusion of outer cortical nephrons fell more with age than did perfusion of the corticomedullary nephrons. Whether this selective decrease in cortical nephron perfusion was due to sclerotic changes in the small arcuate arterioles or represented a selective vasoconstriction of the more peripheral vessels was investigated. The vasodilator acetylcholine increased renal blood flow in both young and old subjects but the effect was more striking in the younger subjects. In contrast, the vasoconstrictive response to angiotensin was similar in the young and old subjects. Modification of sodium intake also produced a striking change in the relationship between age and renal hemodynamics. In young subjects renal blood flow was considerably higher on a high salt diet than on a low salt diet; while in older subjects, renal blood flow was unaltered by the level of sodium intake. These studies suggest that the kidney in the aged patient is in a relatively greater state of base line vasodilatation or else has less capacity to vasodilate than does the kidney of the younger patient.

These data which suggest that aged kidney is in a relative state of vasodilatation are in contrast to those published by Davies and Shock (1950) which suggest a state of resting vasoconstriction in the older patient. Unfortunately no third study exists to resolve this question.

3. <u>Maximum Tubular Transport Capacity</u>. The tubular maximum of PAH or diodrast (Tm_{PAH} or $Tm_{Diodrast}$) is a measure of the ability of the renal tubules to secrete dye when the arterial blood level is raised sufficiently to saturate the tubular transport capacity so that all of the PAH cannot be removed from the blood in one passage through the kidney. The decrease in Tm_{PAH} with age was almost identical to the decrease in inulin clearance observed with age (Davies and Shock, 1950).

Similarly, Miller <u>et al</u>. (1952) observed a decrease in the tubular maximum of glucose ($Tm_{glucose}$) with age that closely paralleled the decrease in inulin clearance with age.

Similar data in patients with various renal diseases led Bricker <u>et al</u>. (1960) to develop their "intact nephron hypothesis". They suggested that as renal function decreased, regardless of underlying cause, surviving nephrons either functioned normally or did not contribute significantly to final urine formation. Their studies demonstrated that as glomerular function declined, there was a proportional decrease in a variety of tubular functions. After Biber <u>et al</u>. (1968) showed by micropuncture studies that damaged nephrons do contribute significantly to urine formation, Bricker (1969) revised his original hypothesis by emphasizing that, despite impairment in glomerular and tubular functions in individual nephrons and nephron segments due to structural damage, the remaining intact, normal nephrons or nephron segments adapted or compensated appropriately to maintain the constant internal environment necessary for the individual to survive.

Although most of the reduction in the secretory and resorptive tubular maximums of the kidney with age may be explained by a progressive loss of nephrons, experiments in rats have shown that there are fewer energy producing mitochondria (Barrows et al., 1960), lower enzyme concentrations (Barrows et al., 1960), lower concentrations of sodium-potassium-activated ATPase activity (Beauchene et al., 1965), and diminished tubular transport (Beauchene et al., 1965) in old compared to young kidneys. Thus, multiple mechanisms of aging appear to exist which include not only changes in the nephron population but changes in basic mechanisms at the cellular level.

4. Concentrating and Diluting Ability. Several studies (Lindeman et al., 1960; Miller and Shock, 1953; Lindeman et al., 1966) have shown a decrease in concentrating ability, as measured by maximum urine osmolality, with age. In one of these studies (Lindeman et al., 1966), maximum diluting ability, as measured by minimum urine osmolality achieved, similarly was decreased with age. One must be careful in interpreting these data, however.

In older persons, total solute excretion should be nearly the same as in younger persons if they are ingesting a similar diet. Actually, older persons do have some decrease in total solute excretion but it is much less than the decrease in glomerular filtration rate with age. This means each surviving nephron in the elderly person is exposed to an increased solute load. Even if all surviving nephrons were completely normal, the solute diuresis per nephron would decrease the ability of the kidney to develop maximal and minimal osmolalities when dehydrated or hydrated respectively. In order to compare concentrating and diluting abilities in young and old subjects, it would be necessary to determine these functions when solute excretion per nephron is comparable.

Another way to compare concentrating and diluting abilities in young vs. old persons would be to compare negative free water clearance ($T^c_{H_2O}$) and free water clearance (C_{H_2O}) respectively corrected for nephron mass as follows:

$$\frac{T^c_{H_2O} \times 100}{\text{Observed GFR}} = T^c_{H_2O}/100 \text{ ml GFR}$$

$$\frac{C_{H_2O} \times 100}{\text{Observed GFR}} = C_{H_2O}/100 \text{ ml GFR}$$

The data in Table II have been abstracted from one of our previous publications (Lindeman et al., 1966) to show that diluting capacity is not decreased with age.

Table II

Maximum Diluting Capacity in Young, Middle-Age and Elderly Male Subjects after Ingestion of 20 cc H_2O/Kg Body Weight*

	Young	Middle-Age	Old
No. of subjects	7	7	7
Mean age (yr)	31	60	84
Mean GFR (cc/min)	149 ± 9	92 ± 8	65 ± 4
Urine flow (cc/min)	19.8 ± 1.7	11.1 ± 1.5	8.5 ± 1.2
Urine osmolality (mOSM/L)	52 ± 3	74 ± 6	92 ± 11
Total solute excretion/100 ml GFR	690	840	1120
C_{H_2O} (cc/min)	16.2 ± 1.4	8.4 ± 1.3	5.9 ± 1.0
C_{H_2O}/100 ml GFR (cc/min)	10.9	9.1	9.1

*From Lindeman et al., 1966.

The impaired ability to form a dilute urine in older persons appears to be attributable to the increased solute load per nephron. When C_{H_2O} is corrected for GFR (C_{H_2O}/GFR x 100) and solute excretion, a normal value is obtained. Minimal urinary osmolality also becomes normal when corrected for solute excretion per nephron.

Similarly, the impaired concentrating ability may be attributed to the increased solute excretion per nephron. The data in the literature now are not available to determine this definitively. However, it is known that elderly persons do respond normally to submaximal graded doses of antidiuretic hormone (Pitressin®) (Lindeman et al., 1966).

5. **Ability to Acidify Urine**. Despite the decrease in renal function with age, the pH, pCO_2 and bicarbonate concentrations in blood of aged persons without renal disease do not differ from the values observed in young subjects in the basal state (Shock and Yiengst, 1950; Adler et al., 1968). The decreases in pH and bicarbonate concentrations of blood were prolonged in elderly persons after ingestion of an acid load, however (Shock and Yiengst, 1948; Hilton et al., 1955).

Table III tabulates the data on three separate age groups of normal subjects studied in 1968 (Adler et al., 1968). After base line studies to define acid-base status of urine and blood, each patient ingested 0.1 Gm ammonium chloride per Kg body weight and serial blood and urine samples were collected over the next 8 hours. The mean decrease in serum bicarbonate concentrations (4.6-4.8 mEq/L) was nearly identical in all three age groups. The minimum urine pH achieved in each age group also was nearly equal.

Table III

Mean $\pm$ S.D. Inulin Clearance, Minimum Urine pH and Measures of Acid Excretion in Response to a Standardized Acid Load (0.1 Gm NH_4Cl per Kg Body Weight) in Three Groups of Normal Subjects of Varying Ages *

	Young	Middle-Age	Old
No. of subjects	10	7	9
Age range (yr)	17-35	49-67	72-93
Inulin clearance (cc/min)	115 $\pm$ 16	95 $\pm$ 12	55 $\pm$ 18
Minimum urine pH	4.96	4.93	4.85
Total acid excretion (8 hr)# (μEq/min)	100		39
Total acid excretion /100cc/min GFR (μEq/min)	78		86
Percent of acid load excreted (8 hr)	35 $\pm$ 6	30 $\pm$ 7	18 $\pm$ 5
Percent of total acid excreted as NH_4^+	72 $\pm$ 7	67 $\pm$ 6	59 $\pm$ 5

*From Adler et al., 1968.
#Total acid excretion=ammonium+titratable acid-bicarbonate

A much larger percentage of the ingested acid load as
measured by total acid excretion (ammonium plus titratable
acid minus bicarbonate) was excreted by the young subjects
(35%) than by the aged subjects (18%). If one factors total
acid excretion by glomerular filtration rate, very similar
values are obtained for the three groups as shown in
figure 2. The young subjects excreted a greater percent of
their total acid as NH_4^+ than did the old subjects. This is
at least partially due to the fact that there was an increase
in urinary buffers making up titratable acid (phosphate,
creatinine, etc.) per unit glomerular filtration rate in the
older subjects.

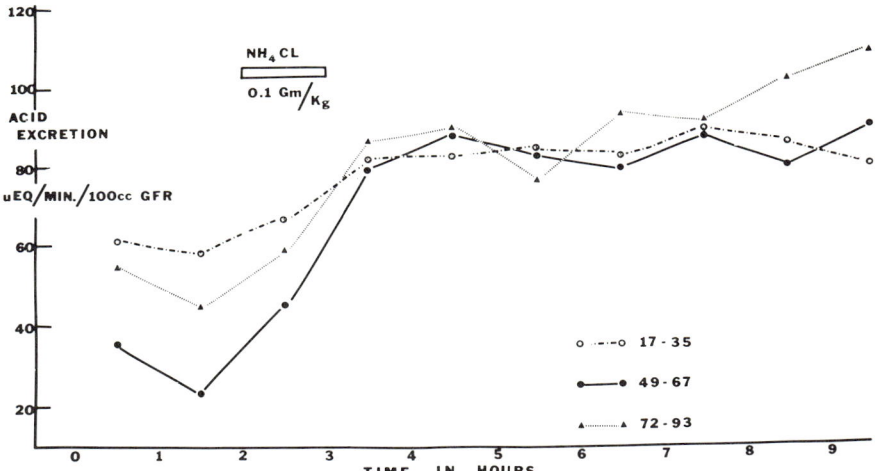

Fig. 2 Mean ($\pm$ S.E.M.) total acid excretion (μEq/min
per 100 ml GFR) in young, middle-aged and old subjects 2 hours
before and 8 hours after ingestion of 0.1 Gm per Kg of
ammonium chloride (Adler et al., 1968).

6. <u>Glomerular Permeability</u>. Little information is
available on the changes in urinary protein excretion with
age. Van Zonneveld (1959), in a population survey involving
over 3000 persons over age 65 years, found an increasing
incidence of proteinuria with age. Still, by age 85, only
32% of his subjects had proteinuria. Lowenstein et al.
(1961) studied glomerular clearance of free hemoglobin in
47 healthy adult males, age 20 to 90 years, free of clinical
renal disease. When free hemoglobin clearance was factored

by inulin clearance, no evidence of an alteration in glomerular permeability with age was present.

Pathophysiology of the Aging Kidney

One of the major unanswered questions remains "How does kidney function decline with age in the individual person?" As shown in figure 3, taking data from previous studies (Davies and Shock, 1950; Wesson, 1969; unpublished observations), utilizing cross-sectional and longitudinal data collected from "normal" aging populations, there is a decrease in mean renal function with age in each decade which accelerates with advancing age. Is this a progressive physiological or involutional change with loss of nephron units systematically through the life of the individual or does renal function remain stable until some pathologic process causes an acute decrease in renal function perhaps with decreasing ability to regenerate or replace injured or destroyed nephrons or cells? If the first were true, then renal function in individual subjects followed longitudinally would follow the dotted line in this figure. On the other hand, some of the types of acute renal injury which might produce decreases in renal function are shown in figure 3 and include undetected glomerulonephritis due to immunological injury, pyelonephritis due to bacterial or viral infections, acute tubular injury or interstitial nephritis induced by drugs, poisons or acute illness, vascular occlusions, and obstruction. Many of these episodes might well go unrecognized as no easy diagnostic tests are available for many of them. Up to age 40, the ability of the individual to regenerate or restore injured nephrons or cells probably remains good; after age 40, there very likely is a decrease in this ability to replace injured cells.

McKay et al. (1932) were the first to document that the aging kidney loses its capacity to replace or regenerate injured or destroyed renal cells. They found that, after unilateral nephrectomy performed in rats aged 30, 60, 270, 360 and 540 days, the hypertrophy of the remaining kidney was 44, 35, 33, 23 and 23% of control kidney weight. Kennedy (1958) subsequently reported differences in DNA, RNA and total nitrogen concentrations in surviving kidneys two to six weeks after unilateral nephrectomy in rats of different ages. He showed that in young animals (one month old), there was striking hyperplasia (an increase in nuclei as indicated by increased DNA content) and hypertrophy (an increase in cytoplasm as indicated by increased RNA content). In old rats (6-months old), there was no hyperplasia and hypertrophy was decreased compared to young rats. The most elaborate studies have been reported by Phillips and Leong (1967) and support these previous observations. They measured the rates of DNA synthesis with tritiated thymidine autoradiography and quantitated mitotic activity in the remaining kidney of young and old rats after unilateral nephrectomy. In both groups, peak incorporation occurred 36 hours after nephrectomy being three times higher in the young as compared to old rats. Although quantitatively the type of response indicative of compensatory hypertrophy is similar in young and old animals, quantitatively the proliferative activity is greatly decreased in the adult animals.

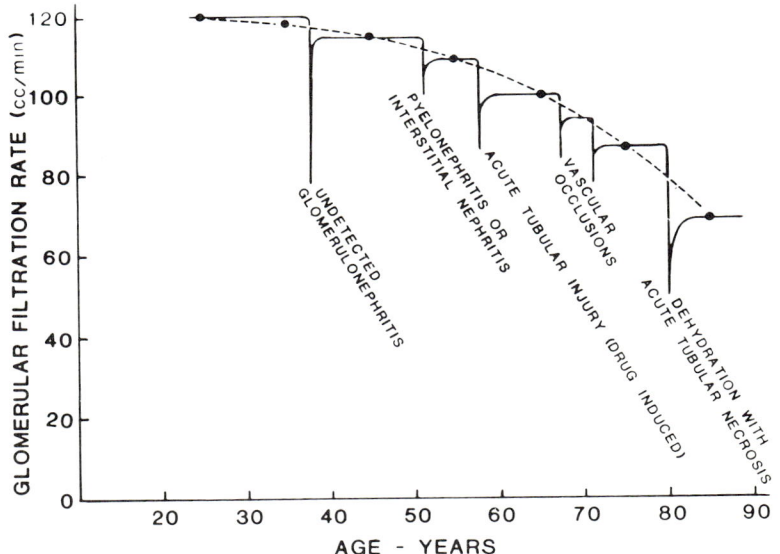

Fig. 3   Mean glomerular filtration rates as determined by cross-sectional studies plotted against age. Whether the kidney ages by a steady progressive involutional decrease in renal function (dashed line) or whether renal function remains stable until some pathological process intervenes with incomplete recovery (solid line) remains undetermined.

A study by Friedman et al. (1972) utilized scintillation scanning techniques to localize defects in kidney function in elderly persons with no past history of renal disease. They found abnormal scans in 25 of 35 elderly patients (71%) with a mean age of 75 years (range 60-93 years) and mean creatinine clearance of 53 cc/minute.

Sixteen (46%) showed focal areas of diminished uptake which were felt to represent ischemic lesions with reduced tubular function. Significant pyuria was present in 37% of the patients, nevertheless, intravenous pyelograms were interpreted as normal in all cases. No significant proteinuria was detected in any patient. These findings are consistent with the hypothesis that focal ischemic lesions due to arteriole occlusions and/or pyelonephritis are contributing in an intermittent pattern to the decrease in renal function observed in individual aging persons.

Tauchi et al. (1971) compared postmortem renal pathology in elderly Caucasians and Japanese. They found arteriosclerotic lesions in the middle and small sized arteries earlier and they were more severe in the Japanese consistent with the increased severity of atherosclerotic disease generally observed in this population. Kidney weight, size of glomeruli, number of cells per glomerular tuft and number of epithelial cells in convoluted tubules in a given area all decreased significantly with age and the decline was significantly more rapid in the Japanese. The size of the individual epithelial cell nuclei however increased significantly with age with the increase more apparent in the Caucasians. The authors concluded that sclerotic and fibrotic changes in the renal arteries paralleling a generalized arteriosclerotic process were responsible for many of the senile changes occurring in the kidney.

Asymptomatic bacteriuria also may be an important contributor to the decrease in renal function with age observed in cross-sectional studies. Dontas et al. (1968) found 24 of 90 clinically healthy residents of the Athens Home for the Aged (27%) had persistent bacteriuria, i.e. greater than 100,000 bacteria per ml. The mean inulin clearance was significantly lower (70 vs. 81 cc/min) in the bacteriuric group when compared to the other residents. The decreases in other measures of renal function (Tm_{PAH} and vasopressin concentrating ability) were even more striking in the bacteriuric residents.

Wolfson et al. (1965) found asymptomatic bacteriuria in 15% of 521 geriatric male patients (median age 63 years). The age-related incidence of bacteriuria was relatively constant at 9% up to age 60 years; it then increased rapidly reaching 42% in individuals over age 80 years. Although the incidence of prostatic hypertrophy, urinary calculi, previous infection, instrumentation and surgery increased with age, there was a significant number of individuals in whom these predisposing conditions were not found.

In order to determine just how the kidney ages in the individual subject, one would need to follow frequently serial accurate and precise measures of renal function in individual subjects longitudinally over a period of many years. Studies have been underway at the Gerontology Research Institute at Baltimore City Hospitals (Shock, 1967) to follow serial endogenous creatinine clearances in a group of over 500 male subjects at 18 month intervals. Unfortunately, the determination of endogenous creatinine clearance is insufficiently accurate or precise to answer this posed question on how the individual kidney ages. Serial inulin (or I^{125} iothalamate) clearances requiring constant infusions, and much more effort and expense per study, ultimately will be necessary.

There are other aspects of renal pathophysiology with aging which have been only superficially explored. For example, the diurnal variations in urine sodium, chloride and potassium excretions and glomerular filtration rate appear to be blunted in older subjects when compared to young subjects (Lobban and Tredie, 1967; unpublished observations). One potential explanation might be that the normal daytime increases in electrolyte excretions and glomerular filtration rate might be partially eliminated by an exaggerated effect of posture assuming that older persons decrease electrolyte excretion and glomerular filtration rate more with standing than do young persons.

Actually when the response to tilt is compared in young and old subjects (Table IV) (Lee et al., 1966), there is little difference in the percent change in sodium excretion or glomerular filtration rate at the end of one hour of tilting, i.e. there is no exaggerated response to tilt when aged subjects are placed in an upright position (figure 4).

Although the effect of age on the renal responses to vasoconstrictors and vasodilators has been determined following glomerular filtration rate and renal plasma flow (Davies and Shock, 1950), little information is available on the ability of the aging kidney to regulate sodium excretion in response to volume expansion and contraction. Elderly male subjects are more likely to develop an exaggerated natriuresis with a water load than are young males (Lindeman et al., 1970). Schalekamp et al. (1971) found that older hypertensive patients, in whom renal vascular resistance and filtration fraction were elevated and plasma renin was suppressed, consistently developed a more marked natriuresis following an intravenous saline load than did young hypertensive patients. The aged individual can conserve sodium under conditions of acute dehydration (Sporn et al., 1962), but how efficiently this is accomplished remains undefined. Furthermore, the ability to eliminate large quantities of sodium when stressed with excessive salt intake remains unknown.

Table IV

Effect of One Hour of 45° Head-Up Tilt on Sodium Excretion and Glomerular Filtration Rate in Young vs. Old Normal Male Subjects*

	Young	Old
No. of subjects	14	12
Mean age (range)	24 (19-34)	64 (47-82)
Supine		
Mean inulin clearance (cc/min)	131 ± 7	81 ± 7
Mean sodium excretion (μEq/min)	200 ± 33	145 ± 26
45° Tilt (60 minutes)		
Mean inulin clearance (cc/min)	111 ± 5	70 ± 7
Percent decrease	15	14
Mean sodium excretion (μEq/min)	82 ± 14	54 ± 7
Percent decrease	59	63

*From Lee et al., 1966.

As stated initially, the kidneys are responsible for maintenance of a constant internal environment of fluid volume and electrolyte concentrations. Imbalances result not from intrinsic renal changes with age, but rather from extrarenal pathology affecting renal regulatory mechanisms, e.g. a change in endocrine balance with age. Figure 5 plots total blood volumes and plasma volumes against age in a large number of male subjects, age 20 to 90 years (Cohn and Shock, 1949). It is apparent there is no change with age.

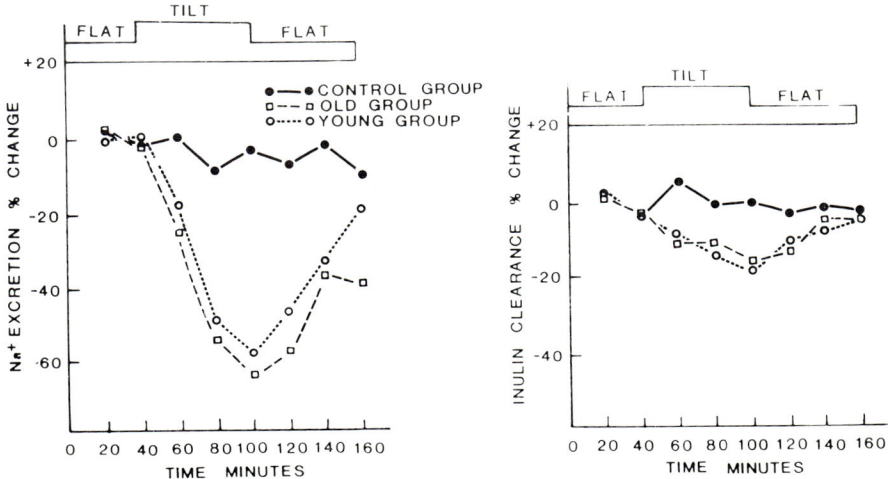

Fig. 4   Effect of one hour of 45° head-up tilt on glomerular filtration rate and urinary sodium excretion in young and old subjects (Lee et al., 1966).

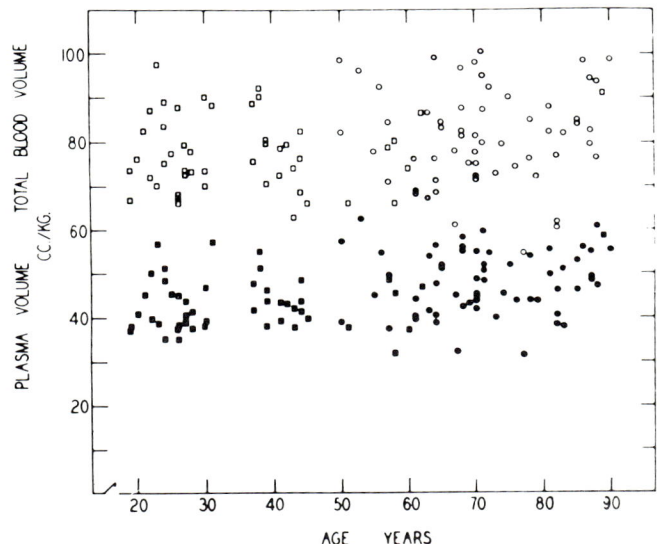

Fig. 5   Total blood volume and plasma volume plotted against age in normal male subjects, age 20 to 90 years (Cohn and Shock, 1949).

Figure 6 shows that extracellular fluid volumes, as measured by determining thiocyanate spaces, also fails to change with age (Shock, 1956).

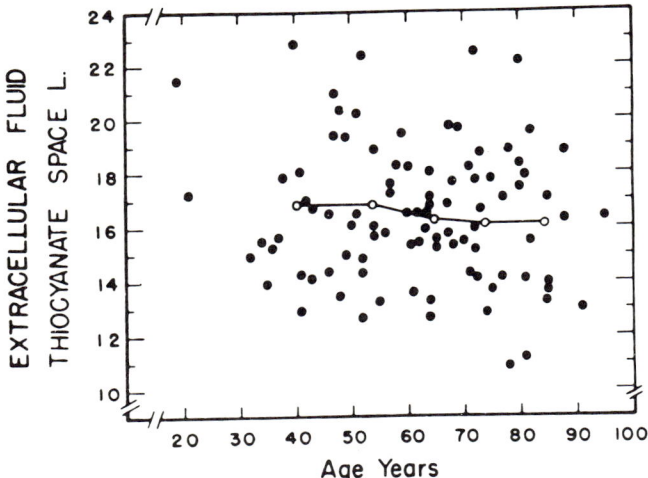

Fig. 6 Extracellular fluid volume (thiocyanate space) plotted against age in normal male subjects (Shock, 1956).

Sodium, potassium, chloride, calcium and magnesium levels are not significantly altered with age under basal conditions (Elkinton and Danowski, 1955; Shock, 1961; Korenchevsky, 1961). Acid-base balance, as discussed earlier, also fails to be affected by age.

Statistically significant changes in the serum concentrations of some of the trace metals have been observed with age. For example, serum zinc concentrations decrease significantly with age (figure 7) (Lindeman et al., 1971), and serum copper concentrations increase significantly with age in the male subjects (figure 8) (Yunice et al., 1974). The etiology and importance of these changes with age remain undetermined but they may well be related to the levels of metal-binding proteins in the serum. It is doubtful that the changes are related to any intrinsic renal alteration with age.

To summarize, the decrease in each of the major functions of the kidney parallels the decrease in glomerular filtration rate suggesting that the major way that the kidney ages is by reduction in the number of functioning nephron units. If there are selective tubular defects, the remaining normal nephrons and nephron segments compensate or adapt to maintain a normal internal environment of fluid balance, electrolyte concentrations and acid-base balance.

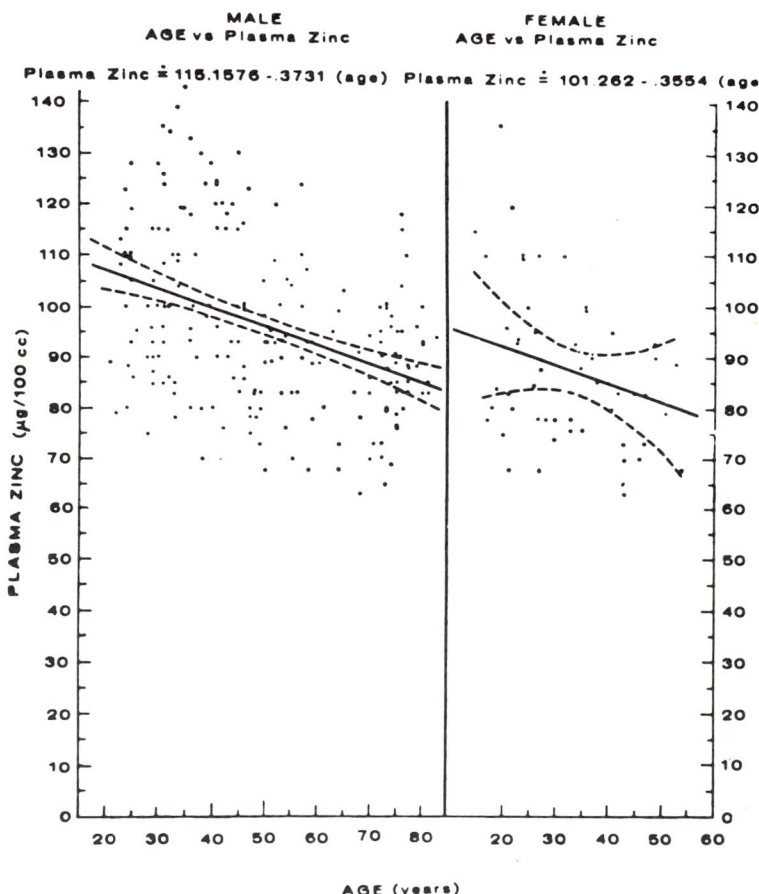

Fig. 7   Plasma zinc concentrations are plotted against age in 204 male and 54 female subjects. The regression line and 95% of confidence limits are shown (Lindeman et al., 1971).

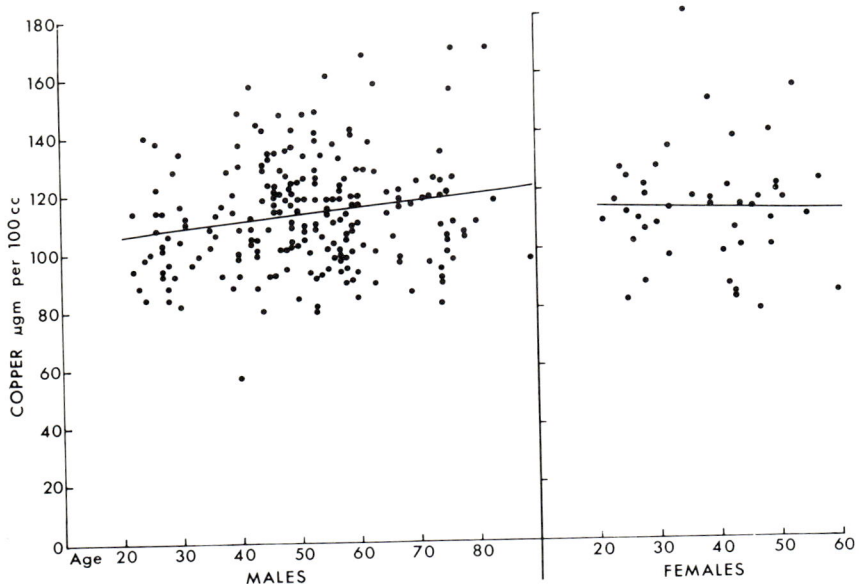

Fig. 8 Serum copper concentrations are plotted against age in 180 male and 44 female subjects. The solid lines are the calculated regression lines (Yunice et al., 1974).

REFERENCES

Adler, S., Lindeman, R. D., Yiengst, M. J., Beard, E., and Shock, N. W. (1968). J. Lab. Clin. Med. 72, 278.
Barrows, C. H., Jr., Falzone, J. A., Jr., and Shock, N. W. (1960). J. Gerontol. 15, 130.
Beauchene, R. E., Fanestil, D. D., and Barrows, C. H. (1965). J. Gerontol. 20, 306.
Biber, T. U. L., Mylle, M., Baines, A. D., Gottshalk, C. W., Oliver, J. R., and MacDowell, M. C. (1968). Am. J. Med. 44, 664.
Bradley, S. E. (1947). In "Transactions of the First Conference on Factors Regulating Blood Pressure", p.118, Josiah Macy, Jr. Foundation, New York.
Bricker, N. S. (1969). Am. J. Med. 46, 1.
Bricker, N. S., Morrin, P. A. F., and Kime, S. W., Jr. (1960). Am. J. Med. 28, 77.
Cohn, J. E., and Shock, N. W. (1949). Am. J. Med. Sci. 217, 388.

Davies, D. F., and Shock, N. W. (1950). J. Clin. Invest. 29, 496.
Dontas, A. S., Papanayiotou, P., Marketos, S. G., and Papanicolaou, N. T. (1968). Clin. Sci. 34, 73.
Elkinton, J. R., and Danowski, T. S. (1955). "The Body Fluids, Basic Physiology and Practical Therapeutics". Williams and Wilkins Co., Baltimore.
Friedman, S. A., Raizner, A. E., Rosen, H., Solomon, N. A., and Sy, W. (1972). Ann. Int. Med. 76, 41.
Hilton, J. G., Goodbody, M. F., Jr., and Kruresi, O. R. (1955). J. Am. Geriat. Soc. 3, 697.
Hollenberg, N. K., Adams, D. F., Solomon, H. S., Rashid, A., Abram, L. A., and Merrill, J. P. (1974). Circulation Res. 34, 309.
Kennedy, G. C. (1958). In "Water and Electrolyte Metabolism in Relation to Age and Sex" (G. E. W. Wolstenholme and M. O'Connor, eds.), pp. 250-263, Little, Brown and Co., Boston.
Korenchevsky, V. (1961). In "Physiological and Pathological Aging" (G. H. Bourne, ed.), pp. 129-144, S. Karger, Basel, Switzerland.
Lee, T. D., Jr., Lindeman, R. D., Yiengst, M. J., and Shock, N. W. (1966). J. Appl. Physiol. 21, 55.
Lindeman, R. D., VanBuren, H. C., and Raisz, L. G. (1960). New Engl. J. Med. 262, 1306.
Lindeman, R. D., Lee, T. D., Jr., Yiengst, M. J., and Shock, N. W. (1966). J. Lab. Clin. Med. 68, 206.
Lindeman, R. D., Adler, S., Yiengst, M. J., and Beard, E. S. (1970). Nephron 7, 289.
Lindeman, R. D., Clark, M. L., and Colmore, J. P. (1971). J. Gerontol. 26, 358.
Lobban, M. C., and Tredie, B. E. (1967). J. Physiol. 188, 48P.
Lowenstein, J., Faulstick, D. A., Yiengst, M. J., and Shock, N. W. (1961). J. Clin. Invest. 40, 1172.
McDonald, R. K., Solomon, D. H., and Shock, N. W. (1951). J. Clin. Invest. 5, 457.
McKay, E. M., McKay, L. L., and Addis, T. (1932). J. Exp. Med. 56, 255.
Miller, J. H., and Shock, N. W. (1953). J. Gerontol. 8, 446.
Miller, J. H., McDonald, R. K., and Shock, N. W. (1952). J. Gerontol. 7, 196.
Phillips, T. L., and Leong, G. F. (1967). Cancer Res. 27, 286.
Schalekamp, M. A. D. M., Krauss, X. H., Schalekamp-Kuyken, M. P. A., Kolsters, G., and Birkenhager, W. H. (1971). Clin. Sci. 41, 219.

Shock, N. W. (1956). Bull. N. Y. Acad. Med. 32, 268.
Shock, N. W. (1961). Ann. Rev. Physiol. 23, 97.
Shock, N. W. (1967). J. Am. Geriat. Soc. 15, 995.
Shock, N. W., and Yiengst, M. J. (1948). Fed. Proc. 7, 114.
Shock, N. W., and Yiengst, M. J. (1950). J. Gerontol. 5, 1.
Sporn, I. N., Lancestremere, R. G., and Papper, S. (1962). New Engl. J. Med. 267, 130.
Tauchi, H., Tsuboi, K., and Okutomi, J. (1971). Gerontologia 17, 87.
Van Zonneveld, R. J. (1959). Gerontol. Clin. 1, 167.
Wesson, L. G., Jr. (1969). In "Physiology of the Human Kidney" (L. G. Wesson, Jr., ed.), pp. 96-108, Grune and Stratton, New York.
Wolfson, S. A., Kalmanson, G. M., Rubini, M. E., and Guze, L. B. (1965). Am. J. Med. Sci. 250, 168.
Yunice, A. A., Lindeman, R. D., Czerwinski, A. W., and Clark, M. L. (1974). J. Gerontol. 29, 277.

BONE-LOSS AND AGING

Stanley M. Garn

Center for Human Growth and Development
The University of Michigan
Ann Arbor, Michigan 48104

As the years go by, there is a decrease in the skeletal mass, involving all (or nearly all) of the bones of the skeleton. The cortex, or more precisely, the compact bone of the tubular or "long" bones diminishes, leaving them more nearly hollow shells. The end-plates of the vertebrae decrease in thickness, reducing their mechanical strength. Cancellous elements decrease in number, leaving relatively few, and those of larger size. The plate-like structures of the vertebrae, the cortical (compact) bone of the ribs, the architecturally complex structures of the vertebrae, the femoral necks and heads, and the articular ends of bones comprising joints are reduced in mass, number and complexity (see figure 1).

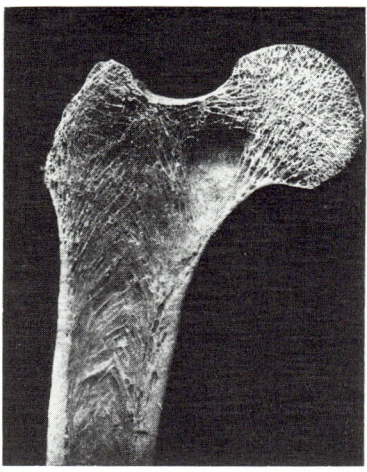

Fig. 1 Adult bone-loss in the femoral head and neck shown in a sawn-section and reproduced from a very early text on aging (Minot, 1908).

The radiologist, observing lesser radiopacity, may describe what he sees as "demineralization", even though both bone mineral and supporting matrix are actually lost. The clinical term "osteoporosis" may be applied, even though the remaining bone is not necessarily more porous, nor spongy or holey. What is lost is not just bone mineral, but bone itself, involving both matrix and mineral. Thus, the bone-loss that occurs in adults with age is bone-loss, relatively pure and somewhat simple. Although adult bone-loss leads to <u>osteopenia</u> and adult bone-loss is what many people mean by <u>adult</u> <u>osteoporosis</u> and <u>senile</u> <u>osteoporosis</u>, it is useful to stick to the simple label adult bone-loss and to search for the reasons why.

THE DIMENSIONS OF THE PROBLEM

Little more than twenty years ago, neither the magnitude of adult bone-loss, nor its prevalence and incidence were known with any degree of certainty. Indeed, at that time, adult bone-loss was then often viewed as a sporadic phenomenon, limited to the postmenopausal female, and it was so named "postmenopausal osteoporosis". Descriptions, now quaint to our ears, made adult bone-loss a unique phenomenon of relatively inactive, postmenopausal, white females, fragile in outer appearance, and given to little consumption of milk or other dairy products.

Two advances in skeletal biology changed all of our thinking about adult bone-loss. The first advance, a milestone in science, is largely attributable to the anatomist-anthropologist Mildred Trotter of Washington University. Weighing dry, defatted skeletons from the Terry Collection of Washington University, and later ashing skeletons, she and her co-workers showed that: 1) skeletal weight decreases with age, 2) it does so in both sexes, 3) skeletal weight decreases in both whites and blacks, and 4) most, if not all bones lose mass with age (Trotter and Peterson, 1955; Broman et al., 1958). Their findings provided the scientific stimulus for most later work on adult bone-loss.

The second advance, involving the radiogrammetric measurement of bone quality, took place simultaneously and independently in several research centers. Christopher Nordin and his group (then in Edinburgh), Richmond Smith, Jr. and his associates (in the Henry Ford Hospital in Detroit) and our group (then at The Fels Research Institute in Yellow Springs, Ohio), all centered particular attention on the cortical and medullary widths of the second metacarpal at midshaft. We sought and we found an approach suitable for large-scale surveys on thousands of living individuals, using available technology and simple caliper micrometry.

Now there are other approaches to in vivo measurements of bone mass, including direct-photon absorptiometry (for which John Cameron and his associates at the University of Wisconsin are largely responsible) and film-type microdensitometry (from Pauline B. Mack and George Vose to Charles Colbert). Detailed analysis made by James S. Arnold of bone mass and bone volume in vertebral sections from cadavers have both confirmed and extended in vivo studies (Table I).

Table I

Approaches to the Measurement of Bone-Loss with Age

Measurement of skeletal weight, ash weight, ash weight to skeletal weight in skeletalized material	Trotter and Peterson, 1955 Broman et al., 1958
Measurement of bone density of vertebral cubes taken from cadavers	Arnold, 1960 Arnold et al., 1966 Arnold, 1970
Direct-photon "densitometry" of the living	Sorenson and Cameron, 1967
Radiogrammetry (caliper measurements of bone shadows on radiographs) of the living	Virtama, 1957 Virtama and Mahonen, 1959 Meema, 1963 Garn et al., 1964 Smith and Walker, 1964 Bonnard, 1968 Garn, 1970 DeQuecker, 1972
Radiogrammetric microdensitometry of film images with or without a reference wedge	Gershon-Cohen et al., 1955 Baker and Schraer, 1958 Colbert et al., 1967

This short diversion into the history of bone-loss knowledge introduces the dimensions of the problem. We now know that adult bone-loss is not limited to the female, rather adult bone-loss takes place in both sexes. Adult bone-loss is not a sudden phenomenon in postmenopausal females; instead it begins a decade or more earlier, and in both men and women. Adult bone-loss is not limited to people of European derivation, nor to any particular racial grouping. Rather, adult bone-loss is a ubiquitous human failing, and from the study of archaeological populations we know that it has long been a major characteristic of aging in man.

THE CONSEQUENCES OF ADULT BONE-LOSS

Since adult bone-loss takes place deep beneath the soft tissues, it is at first scarcely detectable. From the outside there is no immediate hint of the loss of bone tissue at the endosteal surface of tubular bones, nor of thinning of vertebral end-plates, nor of the loss of cancellous structures (especially in the femoral neck). However, as bone mass reduces relative to bone volume, mechanical integrity diminishes. The vertebrae become less resistant to compression, the tubular bones and the femoral neck become less resistant to bending stress. In popular parlance, the bones become "brittle" although in actuality they simply become weaker.

In all individuals beyond a certain age, there is some degree of vertebral collapse and, therefore, stature inevitably diminishes. This is a sudden change rather than a gradual phenomenon, and the age-associated stature decrease is stepwise, as individual vertebrae collapse. With the diminished mass of cortical bone and supporting cancellous structure, the distal radius and ulna and the neck of the femur are expecially vulnerable and so Colles fracture and fracture of the femoral neck are common.

Individual bone-losses have not been related to the probability of fracture, except in the case of some data which we newly possess (Garn et al., unpublished). However, on a group basis, it is rather simple to show how cumulative bone-loss parallels and simulates the cumulative probability of bone fracture (figure 2).

Now the simple Colles fracture is not a major disability. Vertebral collapse and stature reduction is not necessarily debilitating, although associated back pain is discomforting to the point that it has even led some individuals to suicide. Femoral-neck fractures and femoral shaft fractures, however, may be more than discomforting to the aged and so they may be ranked as important, indirect causes of death in the later years.

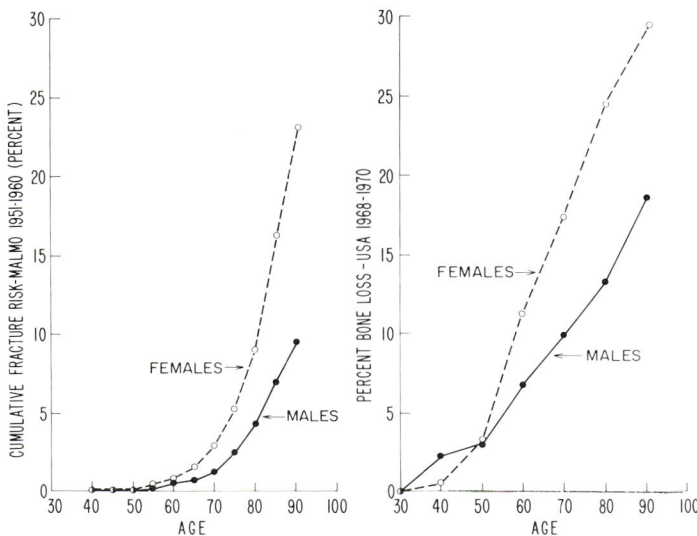

Fig. 2 Cumulative fracture-risk curves (Swedish data, left) and cumulative percent bone-loss curves (USA data, right). Roughly, cumulative percent bone-loss minus 10 equals the cumulative fracture percentage (Garn, 1973a).

SITES OF BONE-LOSS AND GAIN

Now the adult skeletal mass is far from static, both as a repository of mineral, and as a structured entity. The skeletal mass serves as a central bank, with mineral withdrawals taking place during periods of diminished dietary intake, hopefully replaced when intake again improves. Furthermore, there is continual bone remodeling, particularly evident in tubular bones, but with parallels in the round bones and the vertebrae and ribs as well (figure 3).

At the outer (subperiosteal) surface of tubular bones, there is continuing appositional gain lasting through the end of life. This phenomenon of continuing bone expansion, observed early in the skull, was termed hyperostosis cranii by Moore (1955). Later, it was observed in the ribs by Epker et al. (1965) and then well described in a classic paper on the femur by Smith and Frame (1965). With bone expansion in the cranium, femur, metacarpals, rib and vertebrae all documented, continuing bone growth is clearly part of the aging process.

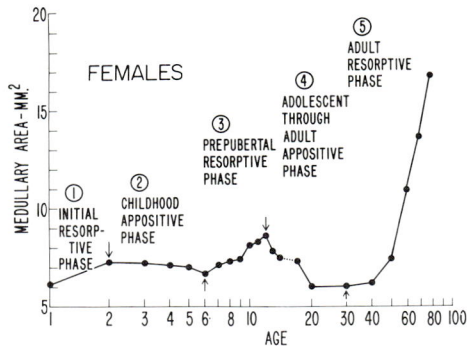

Fig. 3 Phases of bone remodeling at the endosteal surface of a tubular bone, showing the tremendous expansion of medullary cavity area during the adult resorptive phase from the 5th decade on (Garn, 1972, Fig. 2).

At the same time that most bones are getting bigger on the outside, they also reduce in mass from the inside out. In the case of the vertebrae and the round bones, this loss of bone is typically reported as "decreased mineralization", "coarser trabeculation", etc. For tubular bones, the changes are easily demonstrated as endosteal surface resorption, i.e., loss of bone at the inner surface. The medullary cavity gets bigger, the cortical thickness becomes less, and the radiographic appearance is that of lesser "bone" (figure 4).

When femoral "expansion" was first discovered, there was a logical attempt to relate it to weight-bearing, compression-stress and bending-stress, an explanation at least partially tenable for rib expansion as well. When it was later observed that continuing subperiosteal apposition throughout life holds true for the metacarpals and the skull as well, the "use" hypothesis became less tenable. Few of the elderly do hand-stands, and few (except Yoga practitioners and Lewis Carroll's Father William) are spry enough to stand on their heads. A second, alternative "explanation" for continuing bone expansion throughout life is that it has both functional and compensatory value. Outer bone gain, it has been argued, is a natural response (on the part of the bone) to inner bone-loss. However, there are reasons to doubt that gains at the outer surface of ribs, round bones, tubular bones, vertebrae and membranous bones are simple compensatory responses to bone-losses within. Continuing bone growth is essentially linear, from the 3rd decade through at least the 9th. Inner bone-loss begins, as we shall soon show, at the end of the 4th decade, and is maximal during the 5th and 6th decades. What we are describing here are two phenomena, the lifelong small gain at the outer surface and the more precipitous and far larger loss at the inner bone surface and for inner bone.

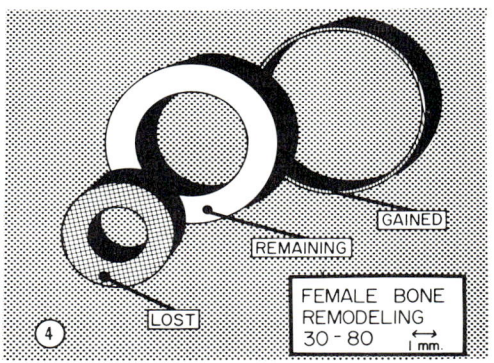

Fig. 4 Age changes at the inner and outer surface of a tubular bone. Contrast the small subperiosteal (outer surface) gain with the larger endosteal (inner surface) loss (Garn, 1970).

THE ONSET OF ADULT BONE-LOSS

Originally, adult bone loss was regarded as essentially postmenopausal, and so attention was directed to women in the 6th, 7th and 8th decades. Trotter's data (Trotter and Peterson, 1955; Broman et al., 1958) suggested an earlier onset, but since her skeletons were limited in number, there were too few individuals to establish the age at onset of adult bone-loss.

It has taken many years and many thousands of radiographs to provide a definitive answer. Bone quality in persons in the 40's is only slightly inferior to that for persons in the 30's, and there is very little longitudinal data beyond that which we described for the period of 1963 to 1970 (Garn, 1970). But with data now available from Central American surveys, and the Ten-State Nutrition Survey of 1968-1970, we can pinpoint adult bone-loss within a five-year period (Garn, 1970). Adult bone-loss, it would appear, begins in the latter part of the 4th decade for the tubular bones of the hand (figure 5). It is certainly not much later than age 40, and certainly not much earlier than age 35. Using curve-fitting techniques the asymptote-age comes out to age 39, the Jack Benny age, which we all remember. Still-limited Cameron-Norland (Mazess and Cameron, 1973) standards (using mid-decade midpoints) suggest a similar age of onset of adult bone-loss, and Arnold's (Arnold et al., 1966) vertebral data also suggest the late 30's as the beginning of bone-loss in both sexes.

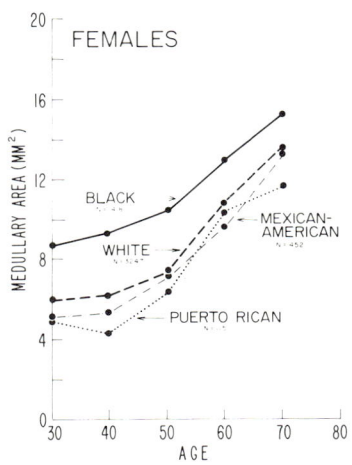

Fig. 5 Adult bone-loss in four populations studied in the USA, showing similarities in the age at onset of medullary cavity expansion (Garn, 1973, Fig. 2).

Whether all bones lose mass beginning at age 39 is not clear, since tibial bone-loss has been observed at slightly earlier ages. Whether all individuals begin to lose bone at the 39th birthday is again not clear, and it will take much longitudinal data to resolve this question. However, it is demonstrable that midpoint age 40 is the turning point in both sexes, and individuals in their 40's have less bone than those in their 30's, despite continuing subperiosteal apposition.

SEX AND RACE DIFFERENCES IN ADULT BONE-LOSS

Two aspects of bone-loss are of extraordinary interest and practical importance to our knowledge of aging. The first is the sex difference in bone-loss; the second aspect relates to the racial similarities and differences in adult bone-loss.

In all groups studied to date, bone-loss can be shown to occur in both sexes, but it is obviously greater in the female. For most groups, we can report a 25% bone-loss in the female as compared with an approximate 12% long-term bone-loss in the male. Moreover, since the initial sex difference in the skeletal mass is of the order of 3:2 rather than 2:1, it can be seen that the female loses more bone, both on an absolute as well as on a relative basis. Expressed in hard gram figures, the female loses 750 grams of her 3,000 gram skeleton, whereas the male loses only 450 grams of his 4,000 gram skeletal mass over a 30-year period. Indeed, for most geographical races and local races, sex differences in bone-loss, both as regards their onset and their magnitude, are similar. Years ago, we (Garn, 1970) showed that bone-loss and sex differences in bone-loss for the six Central American countries formed a family of curves. However, in comparing blacks and whites in the U.S. with samples numbering into the tens of thousands, we have since observed that black women have a lesser rate of adult bone-loss than white women, as shown in figures 6 and 7. Yet this "sparing" of bone in American black women of largely African ancestry is not extended to the black male, who loses bone much as the white male does, albeit from a slightly larger skeletal mass to start with.

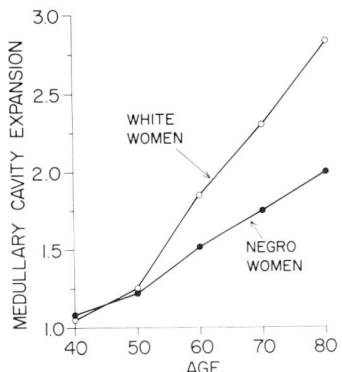

Fig. 6 Comparative bone-loss as indicated by medullary cavity expansion in white women (open circles) and black women aged 40-80. Black women lose less bone both relatively and absolutely. (Data from Ten-State Nutrition Survey, 1968-1970.)

Thus, the lesser bone-loss in the black female, in contrast to all other groups studied, represents a finding of considerable importance. In all groups, adult bone-loss starts at very much the same time, and is far larger in the female than in the male (both on a relative and an absolute basis), but the lesser bone-loss in the American black female represents a departure unique to the black female and not extending to her American black husband.

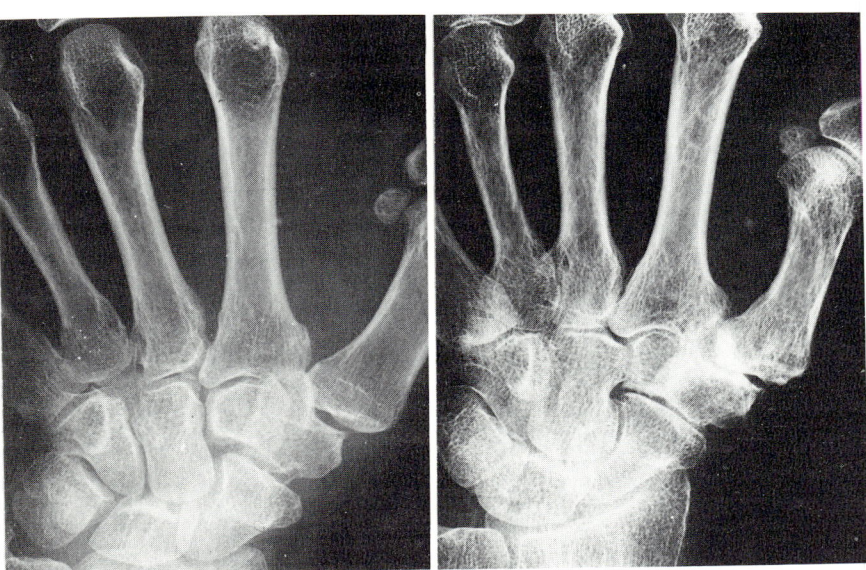

Fig. 7 Comparison of cortical and medullary bone in a black woman (left) and a white woman (right), both octogenarians. Here, as in comparative and tabular data, cortical thickness and cortical area are greater, on the average, in the black female than in her white age-peer, both as the result of more bone to begin with and a lesser rate of endosteal surface resorption.

EXPLANATIONS FOR ADULT BONE-LOSS

Explanations for adult bone-loss have been numerous and varied and some of them simply descriptions rather than explanations proper. In adult bone-loss, some have seen either a reflection of long-term inadequacy of diet or a reflection of decreased activity, while some have adduced hormonal explanations, blaming estrogen, parathyroid hormone, or both (see Table II). Yet other explanations have assumed (a) reduced absorptive efficiency on the part of the aging gut, (b) reduced renal resorption, or (c) increased needs for vitamin D or its more active metabolites. Alternately, loss of bone may be related to the loss of muscle or (arguing from bone-loss in paralysis) that decreased neural impulses lead to loss of muscle and bone together (<u>i.e.</u>, the neurotrophic concept).

Table II

Factors Considered in Relation to Adult Bone-Loss

Variable	References
Fluoride	Leone et al., 1955 Rich and Ensinck, 1961 Bernstein et al., 1966 Garn, 1973b
Altered acid-base balance	Bernstein et al., 1970
Decreased activity	Smith, 1973 Montoye, 1975
Low-calcium intake	Nordin, 1960 Smith and Frame, 1965
Menopause	Meema et al., 1965 Davis et al., 1970
Medullary cavity enlargement	Frame and Nixon, 1970

DIETARY EXPLANATIONS FOR ADULT BONE-LOSS

Since the skeletal mass is necessarily in negative mineral balance during adult bone-loss, early attempts at explanation were directed 1) to calcium and phosphorus intake, 2) to the Ca:P ratio, and, to a lesser extent, 3) to protein intake. Animal studies using rats, cats and dogs variously showed bone-loss in diets low in calcium, low in phosphorus, or with abnormal Ca:P ratios, on diets designed to alter the acid-base balance, and on diets that produced adult protein-calorie malnutrition. Early human studies were directed to a test of the low-calcium hypothesis, since this hypothesis then seemed the most likely.

Studies of older human beings, both on an individual basis and on a population basis have failed to confirm these experimental extrapolations (Garn, 1970). Although bone-loss does result when mineral absorption is reduced (as in postgastrectomy cases), and on diets well below 0.5 gm protein/Kg (as in Indochina prisoners-of-war), there is no present evidence that diet -- within broad limits -- is the predisposing factor in adult bone-loss.

Individuals studied within populations have shown neither more nor less bone, and neither more nor less bone-loss on calcium intakes below 200 mg/day and in excess of 2000 mg/day. Individuals on a low-protein intake diet (below 30 gm/day) have not shown more (or less) bone-loss than those consuming 90-100 grams of quality protein per day. Those who drank much milk and hence have a high Ca:P ratio are neither "protected" against nor exceptionally subject to bone-loss (Garn, 1970).

Population data are equally impressive. Guatemalan natives, low in quality protein intake but with dietaries high in calcium, lose bone at a rate that parallels that of North Americans whose dietary is far higher in protein intake and far lower in calcium intake. Of the many populations studied to date, including those who subsist largely on single-cereal dietaries, there are none who do not lose bone with age. With the single exception of American black women, discussed earlier in this paper, all lose bone at closely parallel rates.

Thus, diet (including dietary mineral and the acid-base balance) does not appear to hold either the explanation or the "cure" for adult bone-loss. While most of us will recommend a dietary reasonably high in calcium, this is done more on hope than evidence. Bone meal may be a useful supplement for the big cats in zoos, but there is no reason to expect bone meal, oyster shell, dolomite chips or calcium gluconate to reverse the 20 mg/day loss of calcium that is the adult negative balance by age 40 or earlier.

HORMONAL EXPLANATIONS FOR ADULT BONE-LOSS

Adult bone-loss, it will be recalled, was once known as "postmenopausal osteoporosis" long before male bone-loss was recognized, and before it became evident that the onset of bone-loss antedates the menopause by a decade or so. Nevertheless, there is evidence that changes in ovarian function do affect the skeletal mass, and this evidence is best adduced from the study of ovariectomized women (see figure 8).

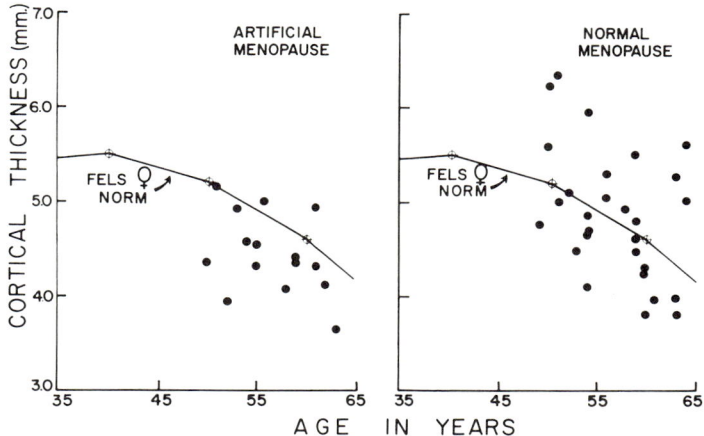

Fig. 8 Diminished cortical cone in ovariectomized women (left) as compared with those who experienced a natural menopause (right) for a comparable age-span. Early ovariectomy results in precipitous bone-loss at the endosteal surface (Garn et al., 1965).

In a general way, early ovariectomy results in an early and precipitous loss of bone at the endosteal surface. The woman who loses ovarian function at 35 shows, by age 45, as little bone as the woman with a normal menopause at age 50 does at age 60. Our interpretation is that, with loss of ovarian estrogens, bone initially added at the endosteal surface is, following menarche, then reduced.

It is impressive, however, that bone-loss goes on long after the bone built at the endosteal surface by action of estrogens is lost. Impressively, bone-loss goes on in the female through ages 70, 80 and 90, losing bone (or more precisely, bone space) originally built 60 or more years before. There is simply more bone-loss, and over a longer period, than the simple estrogen-withdrawal hypothesis accounts for.

In the male, there is bone-loss at the endosteal surface too, beginning at age 39 and continuing until death. Ultimately, the male gets to the point of vertebral collapse, statural shrinkage, and the increased probability of Colles fracture. However, with a 33% greater bone mass to start with, even with a 50% smaller loss rate, it takes him longer. Bone-loss in the adult male poses a greater problem, not so much because of his far lower level of circulating estrogens, but the fact that it takes place at all. In the male, there is rather little post-adolescent bone gain at the endosteal surface. Yet, from age 40 on he loses bone at the endosteal surface nevertheless. The male data, including those for all races, make it less likely that adult bone-loss is simply a phenomenon related to hormone loss.

None of the above relates to whether estrogens or premarin or stilbestrol can long protect the female from adult bone-loss, either following early ovariectomy or normal menopause. Replacement therapy may delay "aging" in other organ systems, as well as in the breasts, the vagina and the apocrine glands. There is scant hard evidence that estrogens reverse or delay aging in the bones (Davis et al., 1970) and even loss evidence that testosterone slows adult bone-loss in the male.

ACTIVITY AND BONE-LOSS

There is notable bone-loss in complete inactivity, unilaterally so in immobilized limbs, unilateral paralyses, and often in amputated stumps, as well. The fact that inactivity, if virtually complete, can result in bone-loss, has raised the question of whether adult bone-loss is a simple reflection of decreasing activity and whether increasing the level of energy expenditure will prevent and even reverse bone-loss in later life.

Now, it is admittedly difficult to provide measures of activity level, for a pedometer does not necessarily measure total energy expenditure. Also, a construction worker may be sedentary off the job, while a desk-ridden executive may engage in greater activity in his leisure off-hours. Nevertheless, some studies on bone quality in individuals characterized by greater activity show evidence of neither less nor of more bone-loss (Montoye, 1975).

There have been attempts to "restore" bone in older individuals by programmed and enforced regimentation or planned activity (Smith, 1973). At least one reports apparent gain, but it is questionable how much real gain of bone is possible in individuals in the 8th decade and above. Similarly, studies of bone quality in athletes and in those who are physically active (such as members of the ski-patrol) may not answer the question, since these individuals may be the result of preselection for muscle mass and skeletal mass, as well.

At present, therefore, it is possible to say that there is advanced bone-loss in virtually total immobilization, but it is not possible to say whether or not various programs of physical activity will prevent bone-loss with age, whether in reference to the total mass or to localized bone-loss. Whether the septuagenarian typist, pianist, cyclist, tennis buff or ski enthusiast loses less bone in hand, leg, arm or spine is not known; however, this information should be obtained. The popular logic that aging effects may be delayed by keeping active is unsubstantiated at least as far as bone-loss is concerned, lacking hard information.

CAN ADULT BONE-LOSS BE PREVENTED?

As with other parameters of aging, there is no certain cure, and no known prevention for adult bone-loss. Rose (1970) is not wrong in asserting that "adult osteoporosis is irreversible" if we add the qualification "as far as we now know". The most that we can surely advocate is having the largest possible skeletal mass to begin with, being male rather than female, and having genes of West African origin.

Present approaches to prevention, including calcium supplementation and moderate doses of fluoride (up to 10 mg/day) are of doubtful and untested efficacy. Heroic dosages of fluoride, up to 60-90 mg/day, along with massive calcium supplementation, may provide symptomatic relief of back pain in advanced cases of adult bone-loss, but the mechanism remains unclear.

Other attempts to prevent or minimize adult bone-loss enters even more into the area of faith rather than certainty. Massive doses of vitamin D, protein supplementation, exercise and premarin all have their advocates, but few proven examples. As of yet, however, other similar age changes such as muscle-loss, the loss of recent memory, leg-pains, or changes in the skin and its appendages cannot reliably be prevented either. For bone-loss in the older adult, the reasonable hope is that methods that may help to restore bone in early adulthood may then be applied to the later years.

ADULT BONE-LOSS AS A MODEL FOR AGING

Despite the manifest disadvantages of adult bone-loss to the individual, which range from decrease in height to loss of life, adult bone-loss also contributes a valuable model for aging research. Few other age-related phenomena are so general, so easily quantified, so simply, in the living individual, using non-hazardous and non-destructive techniques. Few other age-related phenomena are in such a strategic position to help us decide between a unitary and comprehensive theory of aging with all of its implications, and the old wear-and-tear theory that has become the model of this automotive age.

For many aspects of human aging, the way of life constitutes either a large or an undetermined determinant of rate. Adult bone-loss so far and perhaps uniquely, seems independent of major differences in activity, diet, and expectations of aging. The rich and the poor, rural and urban, Londoners and Lacandones all share remarkably similar bone-loss rates when compared with archaeological populations. The bone-loss model thus appears to be a universal model of aging, except perhaps in the region of Lake Rudolph and in southern India.

Some of our colleagues in orthopedics and in mineral metabolism have expressed general disappointment that successive "explanations" for adult bone-loss have come to naught, and that successive attempts at prevention and reversal have been less than universally successful. Rose (1970), as mentioned earlier, expressed his regrets that "osteoporosis appears to be irreversible". Yet if the low-calcium, disturbed acid-base balance, inactivity, low-protein and hormonal-loss explanations seem less than adequate explanations now, let us remember that for most aspects of aging we do not have any operational explanations at all.

Now, the unitary theory of aging includes the assumption that many body systems run down together and that there is a single mechanism that controls them all. It may be that the fibroblasts age, or that there is a neural or hypothalamic clock, or yet even an aging hormone. The bone-loss model allows us to compare loss of bone with declines in other bodily systems, including the skeletal muscle so intimately connected with bone, and with other parameters of aging.

Since bone measurements can be made rather simply in radiographs, we now have age-data on perhaps 100,000 individuals from various parts of the world, with complete life-cycle information on nearly 60,000 persons in our own radiographic collection at the Center for Human Growth and Development in Ann Arbor. In vivo radiography has been so successful as to overshadow cadaver studies, including much-needed analyses of changes in muscle-fiber dimensions which Minot mentioned in 1908. Since caliper micrometry does not measure changes within the bone that remains, it is clear that densitometry (both film-type and direct-photon absorptiometry) must continue, as well as microradiographic techniques using non-screen films and moderate magnification, along the lines that Meema and Meema (Meema, 1963; Meema et al., 1965) have developed.

Now, most studies of adult bone-loss have had as their motivation and their practical purpose the restoration of bone that has been lost, and if not restoration, the slowing-down of bone-loss rates, and if not restoration, the prevention of adult bone-loss. They have not been directed at bone-loss as a part of aging, and at a comprehensive theory of aging. Furthermore, these phenomena have rarely been viewed as the product of not one but several processes, differing in relative importance from individual to individual.

CODA

So let me close with four separate possibilities to explain age-related bone-loss: 1) there is a single, great controlling mechanism of aging that affects bone, muscle, nervous tissue, and other body structures, 2) adult bone-loss is, by contrast, quite independent of other aspects of aging, except for the single dimension of age, 3) adult bone-loss is itself the product of a variety of factors; neural, renal, hormonal and gastrointestinal, and, therefore, differing from individual to individual while concentrated in family lines, and 4) there are a few clusters of aging, mutually independent as clusters, but mutually dependent within.

We have the computer technology to complete the analyses, and we know how to set up the investigative designs to acquire the data. Adult bone-loss may prove to be the very model of aging, or only one model among many, or itself a nesting set of models. Adult bone-loss may confirm: 1) a unitary theory of aging, 2) an additive theory of aging, 3) a parts theory of aging, or 4) it may finally indicate an endless set of aging phenomena, with each individual unique and an example unto himself.

REFERENCES

Arnold, J. S. (1960). Clin. Orthop. 17, 167.
Arnold, J. S. (1970). In "Osteoporosis" (U.S. Barzel, ed.), pp. 80-100, Grune and Stratton, New York.
Arnold, J. S., Bartley, M. H., Tont, S. S., and Jenkins, D. P. (1966). Clin. Orthop. 49, 17.
Baker, P. T., and Schraer, H. (1958). Human Biol. 30, 171.
Bernstein, D. S., Sadowsky, N., Hegsted, D. M., Guri, C. D., and Stare, F. J. (1966). J. Am. Med. Assoc. 198, 85.
Bernstein, D. S., Washman, F., and Hattner, R. S. (1970). In "Osteoporosis" (U.S. Barzel, ed.), pp. 207-216, Grune and Stratton, New York.
Bonnard, G. D. (1968). Helv. Paediat. Acta. 23, 445.
Broman, G. E., Trotter, M., and Peterson, R. R. (1958). Am. J. Phys. Anthropol. 16, 197.

Colbert, C., Spruit, J. J., and Davila, L. R. (1967). *Trans. N.Y. Acad. Sci.* **30**, 271.

Davis, M. E., Lanzel, L. H., and Cox, A. B. (1970). *In* "Osteoporosis" (U.S. Barzel, ed.), pp. 140-149, Grune and Stratton, New York.

DeQuecker, J. (1972). "Bone Loss in Normal and Pathological Conditions". Leuven University Press.

Epker, B. N., Kelin, M., and Frost, H. M. (1965). *Clin. Orthop.* **41**. 198.

Frame, B., and Nixon, R. K., Jr. (1970). *In* "Osteoporosis" (U.S. Barzel, ed.), pp. 238-250, Grune and Stratton, New York.

Garn, S. M. (1970). "The Earlier Gain and the Later Loss of Cortical Bone". Charles C Thomas, Springfield, Illinois.

Garn, S. M. (1972). *Orthop. Clin. North Am.* **3**, 503.

Garn, S. M. (1973a). *Nutrition* **27**, 107.

Garn, S. M. (1973b). "Mineral Nutrition Today". Proc. Miles Symp. 1972.

Garn, S. M., Rohmann, C. G., and Nolan, P. (1964). *In* "Relations of Development and Aging" (J. E. Birren, ed.), pp. 41-61, Charles C Thomas, Springfield, Illinois.

Garn, S. M., Rohmann, C. G., Hull, E. I., and Loxley, M. (1965). "Constituting Progress Report 65-2". The Fels Research Institute (privately printed).

Gershon-Cohen, I., Schraer, H., and Blumberg, N. (1955). *Radiology* **65**, 416.

Leone, N. C., Stevenson, C. A., Hilbish, T. F., and Sosman, M. C. (1955). *Am. J. Roentgenol. Radium Therapy Nucl. Med.* **74**, 874.

Mazess, R. B., and Cameron, J. R. (1973). *In* "International Conference on Bone Mineral Measurement" (R. B. Mazess, ed.), pp. 228-338, Dept. HEW Pub. No. (NIH) 75-683.

Meema, H. E. (1963). *Am. J. Roentgenol. Radium Therapy Nucl. Med.* **89**, 1287.

Meema, H. E., Bunker, M. L., and Meema, S. A. (1965). *Ob. Gyn.* **26**, 333.

Minot, C. S. (1908). "The Problem of Age, Growth and Death". G. P. Putnam's Sons, New York.

Montoye, H. J. (1975). "Physical Activity and Health: An Epidemiologic Study of an Entire Community". Prentice-Hall, Englewood Cliffs, New Jersey.

Moore, S. (1955). *In* "Hyperostosis Cranii", pp. 14-15, Charles C Thomas, Springfield, Illinois.

Nordin, B. E. C. (1960). *Proc. Nutr. Soc.* **19**, 129.

Rich, C., and Ensinck, J. (1961). *Nature* **191**, 184.

Rich, C., and Ivanovich, P. (1965). *Ann. Intern. Med.* **63**, 1069.

Rose, G. A. (1970). In "Osteoporosis" (U.S. Barzel, ed.), pp. 123-132, Grune and Stratton, New York.
Smith, E. L. (1973). In "International Conference on Bone Mineral Measurement" (R. B. Mazess, ed.), p. 397, Dept. HEW Pub. No. (NIH) 75-683.
Smith, R. W., Jr., and Frame, B. (1965). N. Engl. J. Med. 273, 73.
Smith, R. W., Jr., and Walker, R. R. (1964). Science 145, 165.
Sorenson, J. A., and Cameron, J. R. (1967). J. Bone Joint Surg. 49-A, 481.
Trotter, M., and Peterson, R. R. (1955). Anat. Rec. 123, 341.
Virtama, P. (1957). Experientia 13, 236.
Virtama, P., and Mahonen, H. (1959). J. Radiol. 33, 60.

EFFECTS OF HUMAN AGING ON
DRUG ABSORPTION AND METABOLISM

David P. Richey, Ph.D.[*]

Smith, Kline & French Laboratories
Philadelphia, Pennsylvania

The aging human organism experiences a gradual decline in almost all body functions. While most physiological systems continue to perform adequately up to age 60 and beyond, many of these systems do display loss of absolute capacity after age 30. Much of the body's well-being after 30 years of age is due to the large capacity the systems are originally endowed with and to internal homeostatic accommodations. Some of the physiologic declines which occur after age 30 (Shock, 1961) are:

- cardiac performance and output

- renal function

- respiratory function

- lean body mass

- nerve impulse conduction

- muscle strength and tone

- cellular metabolism

- hormonal output

- sensory faculties

- homeostasis

Several of these functional changes may lead to altered drug handling and response in older patients and these are

---
[*]Jointly with A. Douglas Bender, Ph.D.

discussed in detail below.

Age-related changes in drug effects are not solely a problem of the elderly. We emphasize in these comments that the decline of physiological functions even during what may be considered as middle age can lead to an altered drug response. Thus the use of the word "aging" rather than "aged" or "elderly" is most appropriate for this Symposium's focus. A consideration of "Chronologic vs. Physiologic Age in Geriatric Patients" is of no small interest in understanding the importance of individual variations in organ and system senescence, and we commend Dr. Linn's remarks (1975) at this meeting to every student of pharmacotherapy.

The motivation for analyzing the effects of aging on pharmacological response hardly needs explanation. As a group, the elderly experience far more adverse and toxic drug reactions than younger people. With approximately 30 million people over age 65 in the U.S., the elderly constitute therefore a sizable treatment population. Furthermore, the age distribution in this country is increasingly toward the older groups, so that effective guidelines and rationales for geriatric drug therapy is becoming an area of major medical and pharmaceutical importance. Even today there is evidence that a special consideration is required in prescribing for the aged. The approved labeling for many widely prescribed drugs reflects that special concern, although few specifics are offered as dosage guidelines. The emergence of these precautionary instructions and of similar reports in the literature (Bender, 1965a, 1968, 1974; Hall, 1973; Holloway, 1974; Lamy, 1974; Lee, 1972) points to the need for physicians to make some accommodation for age (*i.e.*, "physiologic" age) when prescribing drug therapy (Lamy and Kitler, 1971).

A generalized scheme for pharmacologic action, as illustrated in figure 1, may be of value in considering the basis for these changes in drug response with age. Since most drugs are administered orally, the initial step is their dissolution within the stomach. The drug is then absorbed from the gastrointestinal tract into the circulatory system for distribution to various tissues. The action of the drug will depend on its effective concentration at its intended target tissue, but the concentration of the active drug form will depend on the amount of drug bound by plasma proteins or on the extent to which it is metabolized during its passage through the body.

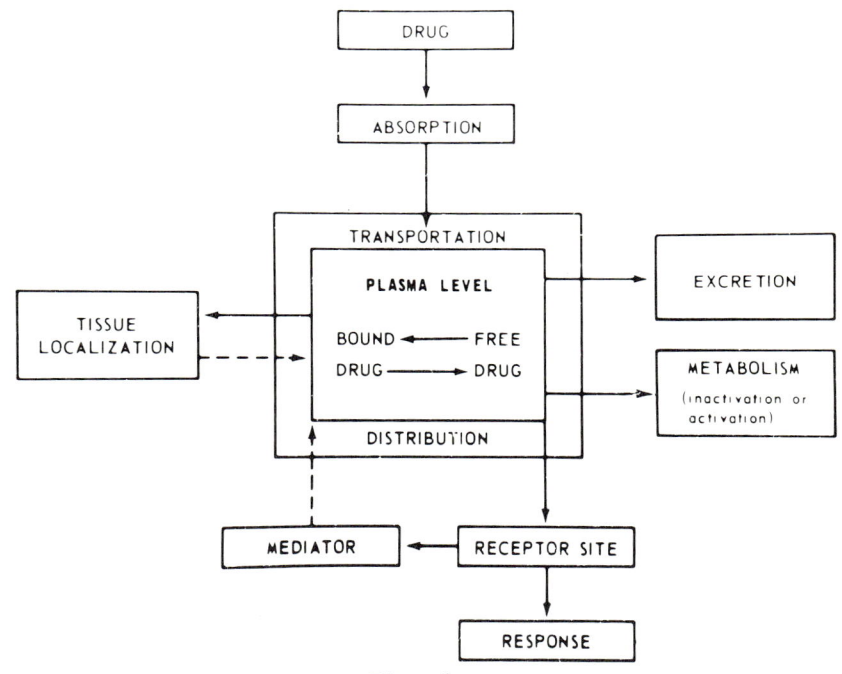

Fig. 1

Primary pharmacologic responses ensue when the drug interacts with a receptor cell or macromolecular receptor, and homeostatic adjustments may follow. The duration of a drug effect will be maximally limited by the rate at which the active form is excreted from the body. The illustration is only a reference framework; not all of the factors enter into the action and handling of every drug. We will discuss later the way(s) in which age-diminished systems affect patient response to pharmacotherapeutic agents.

UNDESIRABLE DRUG EFFECTS

Complications in drug therapy arise when the compound administered is not pharmacologically "clean", that is, when it produces effects other than those for which it is prescribed. The incidence of these undesirable effects may be altered when the action of an administered drug is compromised or potentiated by the presence of another chemical agent or when the organism's physiologic systems are altered from their normal state (as occurs in aging).

Adverse drug reactions (ADR)

In many cases the undesirable side effects associated with some drugs are simply the predictable consequence of that drug's therapeutic ratio (ratio of concentration giving an undesirable physiologic response to that producing the desired pharmacologic effect). Since there is a significant variation among individuals' tissue responsiveness to a given drug concentration, some patients experience an effectively smaller (or negligible) therapeutic ratio and suffer adverse physiologic effects. Reducing the dosage may alleviate the untoward reaction while preserving the desired effect. In other cases, the adverse drug effect is a result of the patient's abnormal handling of the drug and occurs because the active drug concentration at the target tissue (or other tissues) is improper. Altered drug handling may stem from abnormal physiologic behavior of systems depicted in figure 1 and can be genetically inherited or caused by age-associated decrements in tissue function. All of those altered drug reactions (ADR) are pharmacologic in nature, resulting from a pharmacologic response unintended for the drug. Other ADR are of the allergic type, and are either inherited allergies or else have been acquired by sensitization from previous treatment with the drug. The great majority (about 82%) of ADR, however, are pharmacologic reactions (Seidl et al., 1966; Caranasos et al., 1974), and we will restrict our discussion to these cases.

Several studies have demonstrated that the incidence of ADR increases with increasing age. In a prospective study of hospitalized patients, Hurwitz (1969) found that patients over the age of 60 had 2.5 times the number of ADR of those admitted under 60. Figure 2 shows the rate of such reactions as a function of age. Also included in figure 2 are the data of Seidl et al. (1966) from their well-known prospective study in the Johns Hopkins Hospital. Caranasos et al. (1974) found that serious ADR requiring hospitalization also increase with age, approximately doubling in the period from the fifth decade to the eighth decade. All three studies show that women have about twice the ADR incidence of men and that this was exaggerated in white women over 50. More specific reports in the arthritic area indicate that phenylbutazone reactions increase with age by about 30% per decade

(Pemberton, 1954) (see also figure 2) and that gold tolerance decreases with age (DeBosset and Bitter, 1973).

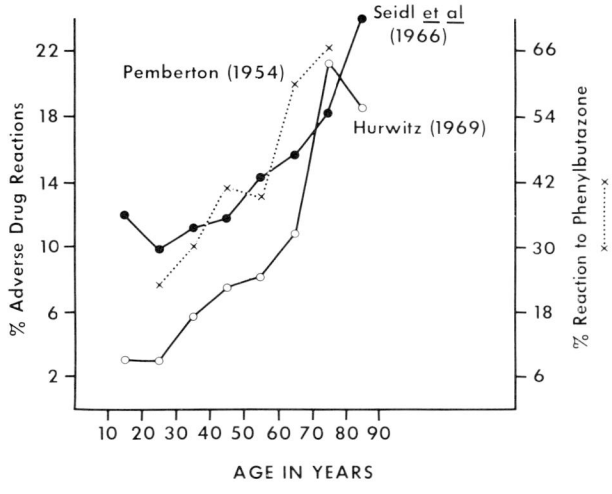

Fig. 2

Psychotropic drugs are heavily used by older age groups, although monoamine oxidase (MAO) inhibitors harbor a serious risk for patients with cardiovascular abnormalities, and tricyclic antidepressants give rise to "central anticholinergic syndrome" more often in the elderly than in the young (Davis et al., 1971). Other ADR common to older patients are presented in Table I.

A factor which we believe to be intimately involved in age-associated ADR is the larger number of drugs taken by older patients. It is axiomatic that older patients take more drugs than younger ones (Lipscomb et al., 1973) yet data relating the average number of drugs taken by different age groups is scarce. Compared to younger people, over-65's spend three times as much for drugs per capita, with an average of 11.4 prescriptions per year versus 4.0 for the younger group (Task Force on Prescription Drugs, 1969). Also if we assume that polypharmacy increases with polypathology, we may estimate the relative drug regimen carried by older patients. A few statistics bearing on the increased pathology of an aging population are that, compared to younger patients, twice as many persons over 65 years of age have chronic disease states and, for those with physically-

Table I

Adverse Drug Reactions of Special Importance to the Aged

Drug	Reaction	Reference
phenylbutazone	peptic ulcer reactivation, hypertension	Pemberton, 1954
MAO inhibitors	dizziness, constipation, hypertension	Witton and Herrman, 1963
benzodiazepines	drowsiness, ataxia	Jones, 1962
cardiac glycosides	anorexia, diarrhea, arrhythmia	Lamy, 1974
levodopa	hypotension, arrhythmia, anxiety	Lee, 1972
hydralazine	headache, angina	Briganti, 1973
tetracyclines	pruritis	Lamy, 1974
aspirin	gastrointestinal bleeding, asthmatic attacks	Briganti, 1973
phenothiazines	drowsiness, confusion, dyskinesia	Ayd, 1961
indomethacin	headache, vertigo, gastrointestinal ulceration	Smith et al., 1966; Lee, 1972
tricyclic antidepressants	arrhythmia, myocardial infarction, hypotension	Janowsky et al., 1974; Weg, 1973
thiazide diuretics	hypokalemia, neural dysfunction, arrhythmia	Weg, 1973 Lamy, 1974
clofibrate	nausea, gallstones	Briganti, 1973
codeine	constipation	Lamy, 1974

disabling diseases, it is 5 times as great. Within the framework of a gynecologic practice, Sotaniemi et al. (1974) found the average number of coexisting diseases (gynecologic plus non-gynecologic) per patient to be 1.3 for the under-30 population, 1.85 for 30-50, and 2.4 for those over 50. In a broader study (Sotaniemi and Palva, 1972), the average number of drugs per patient was found to increase with age, with roughly one-third of those over 60 taking 5 drugs or more. The average number of diseases found in one hospitalized "geriatric" group was 6 per patient, representing usually 4 different etiologic states (Wilson et al., 1962). The distribution mode of polypathology by ages was 3 or fewer diseases for under-65's, gradually increasing to more than 7 after age 80. We can only assume that non-hospitalized patients also show an increase in number of diseases with age, albeit a smaller number than the hospitalized patients, and that their drug regimen increases in parallel fashion. From that standpoint it is interesting that Cluff (1967) and Smith et al. (1966) have reported the number of drugs administered to one patient simultaneously to have a direct bearing on that patient's likelihood of experiencing an adverse reaction. This relationship is illustrated in figure 3.

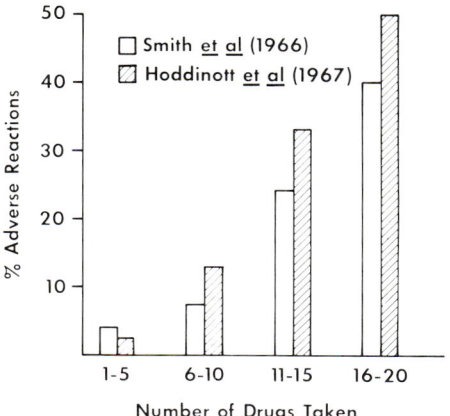

Fig. 3

The data of Hurwitz (1969) support this finding, showing a 3.4% incidence of ADR in patients taking from 1 to 5 drugs and 24.8% in those taking 6 or more. With the large number of medications (both prescribed and over the counter) taken by older patients, there should be little surprise that these patients suffer more ADR. The many published reports of excessive drug regimen discovered in some patients hardly needs citing, as well as the need for every prescribing physician to make a thoughtful evaluation of his patient's drug burden before adding to it. In the absence of any data to distinguish between altered drug handling and excessive drug burden, we can only seek to understand better the former and to minimize the latter.

Drug interactions

Because many commonly used drugs have a pharmacological or chemical effect on physiologic drug-handling systems or on the target tissues of other drugs, there sometimes occurs an interaction between simultaneously administered agents, such that one drug may antagonize or potentiate the action of the other. The exponential rather than linear nature of figure 3 suggests that many ADR are due to drug interactions and this is no doubt a significant component to the age-related side effects shown in figure 2. The relatively large number of drugs taken by older patients makes this group an increased risk for drug interaction problems. Drug interactions may arise at any of the steps illustrated in figure 1, and the age-related changes in these systems make it difficult to predict the extent of such interactions in older patients.

There is abundant literature on drug interactions (Fann, 1973; Morselli et al., 1974; Nies, 1974) and a few of the common interactions pertinent to older patients' drug programs deserve mention. Some detail is warrented in these examples since many of the interactions are due to drug-induced physiologic alterations which resemble age-associated changes in those same physiologic systems. Probably the best known example in the geriatric area is the effect of some diuretics on the action of digitalis toxicity. These are two agents commonly prescribed for edematous patients with congestive heart failure. The action of ethacrynic acid, furosemide, and the thiazide diuretics is to increase urinary potassium (K^+) excretion and decrease serum potassium levels. Since digitalis derivatives depend on K^+ to regulate their cardiac-stabilizing effect, the hypokalemic patient may become very liable to digitalis toxicity.

With reference to figure 1, the digitalis-diuretic interaction involves interference with the mediation step of digitalis action. Other drug interactions may occur at any point in the scheme. At the very beginning of the pharmacotherapeutic process is the matter of drug absorption, and several drug interactions are known to occur which alter this step, usually by reducing the absorption of one or both drugs. Cholestyramine is intended to complex with bile acids but can also bind thyroxine, digitoxin, and other acidic compounds to reduce their soluble concentration. Tetracyclines or phenothiazines may form complexes with antacid components and fail to be absorbed (Nies, 1974). Conversely, antacids may enhance the absorption of basic compounds by raising the gastric pH to allow enhanced membrane-permeability of the nonionized form of the drug. Other alterations of drug absorption may result from administration of agents which change gastrointestinal motility, and we will return to this topic later.

The dosage selected for any drug is intended to maintain a certain effective level of that drug in the body in the face of a characteristic rate of metabolism and excretion of that agent and its metabolites. Most of the metabolism occurs in the liver and it is well known that many drugs can accelerate or inhibit this conversion and thus alter the rate of breakdown of other drugs. For example, phenobarbital or diphenylhydantoin induce higher levels of hepatic enzymes and hasten the metabolism of many drugs, e.g., warfarin, phenothiazines -- diminishing therefore the effect of those drugs. On the other hand, tolbutamide metabolism is inhibited by the presence of chloramphenicol or phenylbutazone or several other drugs (Rowland, 1974), and hypoglycemia may result. An idea of the magnitude of drug-induced metabolic changes may be gathered by realizing that phenobarbital is only one of 60 different drugs reported to increase hepatic drug metabolism and that the metabolism of at least 200 drugs is reported to be altered by phenobarbital. Even within the context of hepatic enzyme inducers, there are complex drug interactions due to differing metabolic rates and affinities of these compounds. While both phenobarbital and diphenylhydantoin raise hepatic enzyme levels, only the former causes accelerated metabolism of antipyrine or pentazocine since diphenylhydantoin competes with and displaces the other drugs from these enzymes -- diphenylhydantoin actually decreases the metabolism of antipyrine and pentazocine, and prolongs their pharmacologic action (Sotaniemi, 1973). Drug interactions also occur as a consequence of altered renal excretion. The effect of probenecid to inhibit penicillin excretion in the renal tubule is well known and may lead to a very high accumulation of penicillin. Phenylbutazone, in addition to

inhibiting the metabolism of tolbutamide, also inhibits the
tubular secretion of acetohexamide metabolites (which also
have hypoglycemic action) (Field et al., 1967) and is therefore contraindicated for both these antidiabetic agents.

An example of drug interaction at the receptor itself
is presented in the use of the antihypertensive drug
guanethidine. In order to exert its effect, this drug must
be transported into sympathetic nerve endings by the
norepinephrine pump, but this process can be blocked by
tricyclic antidepressants. Thus, antihypertensive therapy
will be ineffective if the tricyclics are present, and a
cerebrovascular crisis is a definite risk. Table II lists
a few other drug interations of importance to older patients.

Adverse drug reactions and drug interactions are the
payment exacted for the availability and use of so many
potent therapeutic agents. For a variety of reasons those
complications are more prevalent and aggravated as the
patient grows older. Since there is no question of Medicine
abandoning the available therapeutic compounds because of
these drawbacks, it is imperative that we develop an
effective understanding of the qualitative and quantitative
changes in drug handling and response which accompany the
aging process. We have reviewed the experiemtnal information
which appears to bear on this problem and will present those
data which we feel best enables us to place geriatric
pharmacology within a rational framework.

AGE-ASSOCIATED CHANGES IN DRUG HANDLING

Two issues should be cited here to clarify the purpose,
intent, and scope of this discussion. First, our review of
age-related changes in drug disposition does not imply that
chronologic age per se is the only determinant in considering
a therapeutic regimen, but more importantly stresses that
physiological status is critical to the achievement of the
optimal benefit from drugs. Second, we are not considering
the effect of age on the chemical activity and utility of
specific drugs, only the pharmacodynamic basis for some of
these changes. The guidelines for treatment of specific
disease states and the use of specific agents have been
covered in several excellent reviews (Freeman, 1965; Hall,
1973; Holloway, 1974; Lamy, 1974; Modell, 1974).

We have presented the foregoing material on undesirable
drug effects because they are potentially a major problem in
geriatric pharmacology both as regards efficacy and safety.
We have suggested that these changes often can occur solely
as a result of age-associated changes in physiologic function

Table II

Drug Interactions

Primary Drug	Secondary Drug	Effect on Disposition of Primary Drug
tetracycline aspirin	antacids cholestyramine	decreased absorption due to complex formation
warfarin	phenylbutazone	increased level of free drug due to displacement from plasma proteins
digitoxin	phenobarbital	increased metabolism
diphenylhydantoin	chloramphenicol	decreased metabolism
acetohexamide penicillin	phenylbutazone probenecid	decreased clearance
guanethidine	tricyclic antidepressants	blocked from receptor
digitalis	furosemide, ethacrynic acid, thiazide diuretics	toxicity risk increased due to mediator (K^+) depletion

and that the problem can be compounded by interactions between drugs. The remaining portion of this discussion will examine more closely the basis for these changes in senescence in the therapeutic value and index of drugs.

All of the factors which enter into an organism's interaction with a drug seem to fall into two basic groups -- one group composed of those factors which alter the level of the drug at the target site (absorption, metabolism, plasma binding, distribution, and excretion), and the other group composed of those factors which affect the tissue response to the drug (drug-receptor interaction, mediators, cellular metabolism, and homeostatic mechanisms). The focus of our comments will be limited to absorption, metabolism, and excretion.

Absorption

Deficiencies in gastrointestinal absorption can be a potentially significant factor in therapeutic failures; certainly they have been found to be so in the case of nutritional problems. This is exemplified by the experience of one investigator who reported that several patients suffering from cheilosis showed no response to large oral doses of riboflavin, yet were rapidly relieved by intramuscular (i.m.) administration of riboflavin (Archambault, 1974). Since the solution of this particular case was serendipitous, one can only conjecture on the actual number of absorption failures possibly involved in nutrition and drug therapy.

The entry of a drug into the bloodstream from the gastrointestinal tract occurs in two ways: <u>passive absorption</u>, which involves transient dissolution of the drug in the biologic membranes separating the compartments and which is the major form of drug absorption; and <u>active transport</u>, which involves the translocation of the drug by a stereospecific, macromolecular component located in the membrane.

Earlier reviews on geriatric drug use (Bender, 1968, 1974; Holloway, 1974; Lamy, 1974) have pointed out that there is relatively little information available on age-dependent variations in drug absorption, and this remains true in 1975. The classical reports on nutrient absorption provide the guidelines for these reviews' conclusions, which are as follows. There is a general consensus that the active transport of glucose, galactose, and 3-0-methyl-$\underline{D}$-glucose all show a significant decline with age. These three monosaccharides are all absorbed via a single transport system whose specificity extends to several glucose analogs, but does not include fructose, lactose, or sucrose. Because the active transport mode of absorption requires metabolic energy, glucose transport can be blocked by inhibitors of energy generation, such as dinitrophenol (DNP) or by local ischemia (Robinson et al., 1965). It may be significant also that non-intestinal mammalian cells, whose specific transport systems are not energy-linked, also show age-related decreases in most of their transport capacities, including glucose. These decreases are thought to stem from physical alterations in the cellular membrane (Furcht and Scott, 1973) or to be related to the increased cyclic AMP levels in senescent cells (Sheppard, 1972), and may occur also in cells of the aging intestine. As with almost all compounds transported by specific systems, glucose can enter by passive diffusion also, although at a lower rate. Calcium absorption by the intestine also decreases with age and, like glucose, approaches passively absorbed levels in old animals (Schachter et al., 1960). In this case, the active absorption is known to be catalyzed by a calcium-binding protein whose synthesis is in turn regulated by the active form of vitamin D (Wasserman and Taylor, 1968). Considering the incidence of senile osteoporosis, it seems plausible that the metabolic transformation of vitamin D to its active form is impaired with increasing age and that calcium absorption is similarly impaired.

On the other hand, the absorption of other specifically transported substances such as vitamin B_{12} (Hyams, 1964; Davis et al., 1965), thiamine (Draper, 1958), and most amino acids (Penzes et al., 1968; Penzes, 1970, 1974) are not significantly altered in older subjects. The reviews cited also describe the scattered reports on the absorption of fat, minerals, and other vitamins, but no clear trend is apparent.

Studies more relevant to drug absorption have been reported for xylose and for iron, which are both absorbed passively like drugs. For xylose, it was found that the time course of blood levels achieved by young and by older subjects was fairly similar up through about age 80 (Fikry and Aboul-Wafa, 1965; Guth, 1968) (see figure 4). Beyond age 80, there was observed a significant decrease in the peak blood level, a delay in peak level achievement, and a prolonged decay phase. This was interpreted by the authors to reflect decreased gastrointestinal absorption, and the reduced urinary excretion of xylose by the older subjects seemed to support this. Other studies (Sapp et al., 1964; Pelz et al., 1968) relying on urinary xylose determinations have estimated the reduction in xylose absorption by subjects in their eighth decade to be reduced by 40%. We shall refer once more to these data below, since they are also relevant to the role of renal function in drug therapy.

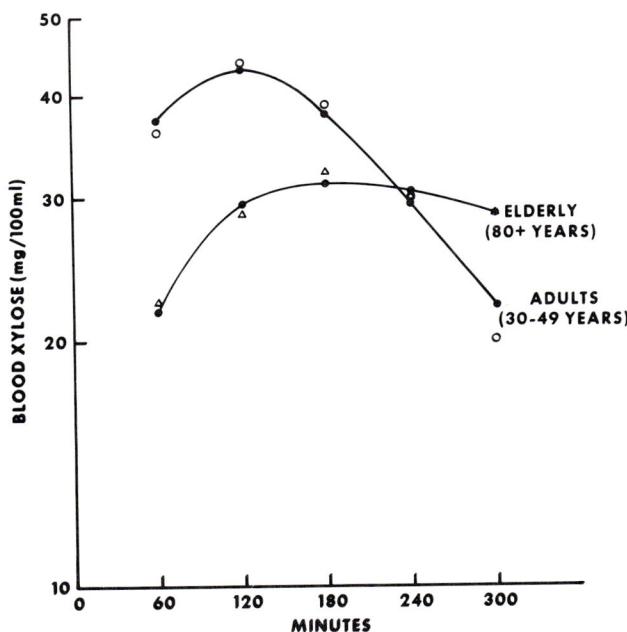

Fig. 4   Time course of blood levels of xylose administered orally. Data from Guth (1968).

The major reasons cited for the reduced absorption were decreased efficiency in the "transport" system, fewer intestinal absorbing cells, and a blood flow decrease due to atherosclerosis but no conclusive evidence was available. In the other example (Dietze et al., 1971), iron administered orally to elderly subjects (avg. age = 79) gave lower blood levels and a decreased peak blood level compared to younger subjects, reminiscent of the xylose curve in older patients (see figure 5). Lower iron absorption was also found in rats of increasing age (Yeh et al., 1965; Jacobs and Owens, 1969). There is no definitive information published to indicate whether lactoferrin is involved in this age-related decrease.

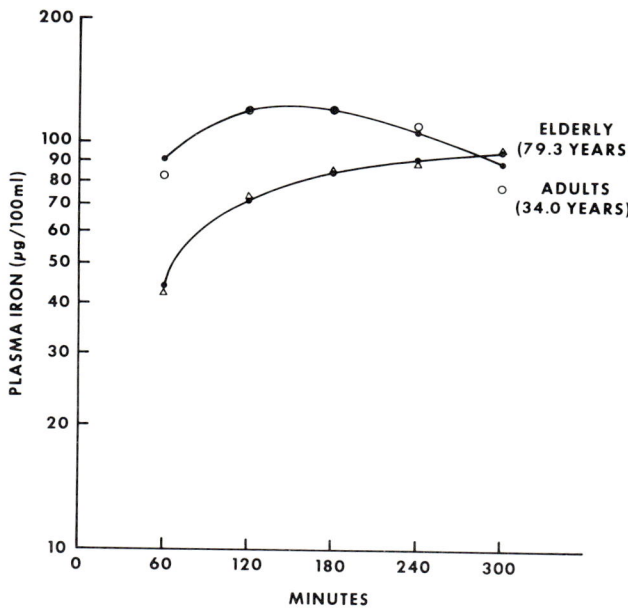

Fig. 5 Time course of blood levels of iron administered orally. Data from Dietze et al. (1971).

Studies on drug absorption rarely include actual age-dependent variability, but there are a few that bear relating. Paracetamol peak blood levels were found to be highly dependent on age (Gwilt et al., 1963), with the highest levels attained by the 35-40 age group and a steep decline for both younger and older subjects. Similarly, penicillin V absorption from the intestine was found to decrease with increasing age in rats over 12 months of age (roughly the onset of rat "middle age") (Niedermuller et al., 1974). Diazepam blood levels have also been reported for subjects of different ages (Garattini et al., 1973). These data show a lower peak level and a longer half-life in elderly subjects (>60 years of age), as illustrated in figure 6.

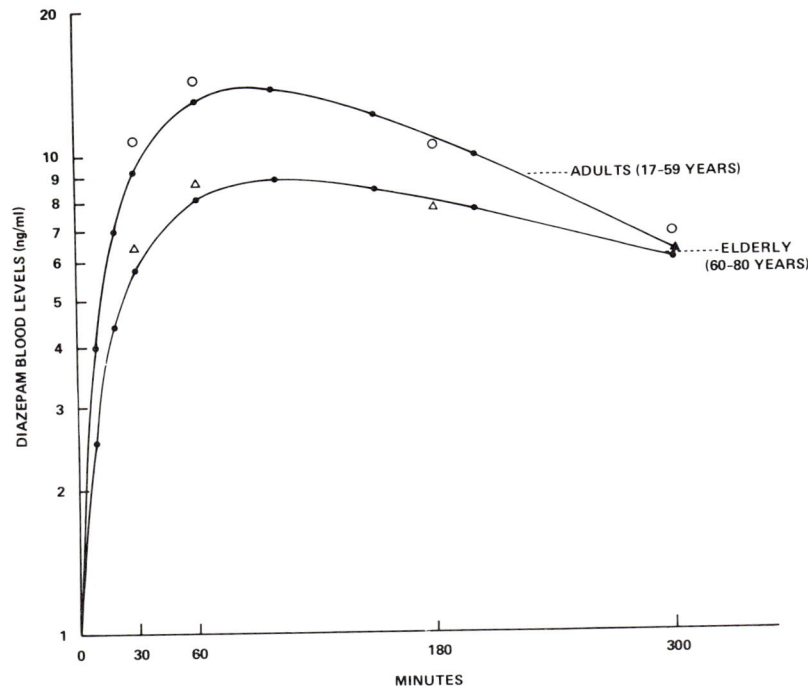

Fig. 6 Time course of blood levels of diazepam administered orally. Data from Garattini et al. (1973).

Because the majority of drug prescriptions are for solid dosage forms to be administered orally, a prime consideration in drug absorption is its solubility in aqueous and organic milieus. Naturally these formulations must render the active ingredient soluble within a reasonable period of time, usually a few hours, in order that it be effectively absorbed by the gastrointestinal mucosa. Remember that with most drugs, absorption will depend on the membrane (lipid) solubility of the particular drug involved.

There is a widespread belief that the drug formulation must be soluble at the very low pH of the stomach in order to permit effective absorption of the drug, and while the formulation solubility is truly important, this general concept is erroneous on two other counts. First of all, the pH of the stomach is not uniformly low; secondly, the stomach is responsible for only a small amount of drug absorption relative to the amount absorbed in the small intestine.

pH

In the matter of gastric pH, it should be recognized that even in individuals with apparently normal stomach acid production, the pH may rise to 7 during the day (Meldrum et al., 1972), especially after eating. The production of stomach acid does decrease with increasing age however (Baron, 1963) and achlorhydria is common in the elderly (Prescott, 1974b), thus leading to the possibility that the average gastric pH is higher in older subjects. Whether a drug be in the stomach or in the small intestine, the local pH will exert an effect on its membrane solubility and thus influence absorption of that drug through the mucosa. Briefly stated, the pH-partition theory holds that any given drug will be more lipid soluble in its non-ionized or in its least-ionized form. It will therefore display its greatest lipid solubility at pH values either above or below its pKa according to whether it is a weakly basic or a weakly acidic compound, respectively. Almost all drugs in common use are either weak acids or weak bases -- mostly weak bases -- and those which have stronger acid-base character are generally poorly absorbed because they are ionized over almost the entire physiological pH range. From a pharmacodynamic standpoint, lipid solubility is represented by an oil/water distribution ratio and is an index of the ability of a compound to be absorbed across cellular (mucosal) membranes. The therapeutic importance of this index is reflected by its considerable employment in mathematical approaches to "drug design". Drug design is a computational approach to correlating an observed biological activity with the measurable physicochemical parameters of a compound eliciting that activity (Hansch and Fujita, 1964; Redl et al., 1974). To date, the partition coefficient is the most widely applicable character useful for predicting the relative biological potency among a series of similar (related) compounds, and this is a direct reflection of the pivotal importance of absorption on chemotherapeutic effectiveness.

Unfortunately, drug solubility and drug absorption have opposite dependencies on pH. Aspirin, for example, is an acid and might be expected to be better absorbed at low pH, yet is insoluble at acid pH (Pottage et al., 1974). Since the majority of organic compounds used as drugs have quite poor aqueous solubility in their non-ionized form, they require an ionizing pH in order to dissolve and thus are presented in a poorly absorbable form. The gastrointestinal pH will determine the rate of dissolution. This problem is frequently circumvented by supplying the drug as a salt which dissolves readily at normal gastrointestinal pH values. Examples of this are sodium salicylate, sodium chlorothiazide, ergotamine tartrate, chlorpheniramine maleate, and the hydrochlorides of ephedrine, dibucaine, hydroxyzine, etc. After dissolution, the drug assumes an ionized/non-ionized ratio according to the environmental pH, and absorption occurs largely in accordance with the pH-partition theory. The gastric pH also affects motility and higher pH values affect absorption by hastening the presentation of the stomach contents to the small intestine.

Absorption in the small intestine

Most drugs being weak bases -- note the large proportion of hydrochloride forms among drugs -- they can be expected to be better absorbed in the small intestine than in the stomach. However, even in cases involving weakly acidic drugs, where the stomach would appear to be a better site for drug absorption than the small intestine by virtue of the stomach's lower pH favoring the non-ionized drug form, the small intestine proves to be the more effective absorbing tissue (Levine, 1970; Prescott, 1974a). This situation evolves simply because the small intestine has an enormously convoluted surface, with folds, villi and microvilli so numerous that its effective surface area is perhaps 2 orders of magnitude larger than that of the stomach, and so may overcome a large difference in _rate_ of absorption. Within the small intestine itself, the mucosal surface area (per unit length) is largest near the top (duodeno-jejunal flexure) and is responsible for much of the drug absorption in the body. The motility in the duodenum and jejunum is rather high however and equal drug may be absorbed in the ileum because of the rather greater length of time the intestinal contents may spend in the ileum (Marcus and Lengemann, 1962). Whichever aspect may be dominant, the small intestine collectively is the major site of drug absorption. It has been found that the total small intestinal mucosal area is directly proportional to body surface area (Wilson, 1967), and this may be the anatomical validation for prescribing dosage on a surface area basis.

Gastrointestinal motility

While in the older patient, the body surface area may sometimes be considered in prescribing dosage, probably less well recognized is the importance of gastrointestinal motility on the absorption of drugs. For example, warfarin (Kekki et al., 1971), barbiturates (Kojima et al., 1971), aspirin (Siurala et al., 1969), and many other drugs are absorbed predominantly in the small intestine, and their rate of absorption overall may ultimately be limited by the rate of gastric emptying. Thus, rapid gastric emptying leads to greater and more rapid drug absorption, which comparably increases or hastens pharmacologic response. Conversely, rapid intestinal motility tends to decrease drug absorption by decreasing the amount of time the drug spends in the area of rapid absorption before being directly voided. An example of a drug preferentially absorbed in the intestine is paracetamol. Heading et al. (1973) found that subjects with a normal gastric emptying half-time (less than 55 min) averaged four times as much paracetamol effectively mobilized as those with slower gastric emptying. Peak blood levels and the rate of absorption of this drug were found to vary inversely with the emptying half-time. Paracetamol absorption in patients with pyloric stenosis was very slow, but was unimpaired in achlorhydric patients (Pottage et al., 1974).

Prescott (1974b) and Levine (1970) have described the effects on drug absorption of several agents which alter gastrointestinal motility. Anticholinergic drugs can decrease the absorption of aspirin or paracetamol (Nimmo et al., 1971) by delaying gastric emptying, and metoclopramide can increase their absorption by stimulating that same action. Agents such as propantheline which prolong intestinal transit time will increase the absorption of aspirin, etc. according to the same rationale. The therapeutic situation becomes very complicated of course when we consider that, in practice, a patient may be simultaneously taking drugs absorbed preferentially in different portions of the GI tract, that some drugs are metabolized to inactive forms in stomach (methyldigoxin or penicillin) or intestine, and that paradoxical absorption may occur for small or sustained release preparations.

The manipulation of gastrointestinal motility is nevertheless a plausible strategy for geriatric and other physicians confronted with a patient exhibiting poor drug absorption; yet it is probably doubtful that we fully appreciate the magnitude of the difference among normal individuals' GI motility, let alone for the aging patient.

An excellent clinical example of inadequate drug absorption was presented by Bianchine et al. (1971) for L-DOPA therapy. Studying the variable success experienced in treating Parkinsonism patients with this agent, they noted that L-DOPA was rapidly metabolized in the stomach (Rivera-Calimlim et al., 1970) and that those patients with longer gastric emptying rates achieved proportionately lower serum L-DOPA levels. They found that one patient whose Parkinsonism symptoms were completely refractory to L-DOPA therapy achieved blood L-DOPA levels only one-third that of responsive patients. Furthermore, this patient had a gastric emptying time of 7 hours, compared to 1 to 2 hours in the successful patients. He had no intestinal absorption defect since he could effectively absorb L-DOPA introduced into the intestine by intubation. When an antacid was administered with L-DOPA, the patient's gastric pH rose from 1.2 to 4, his gastric emptying time decreased to 1 hour, and his serum L-DOPA level rose by a factor of 4. Consequently, his Parkinsonism improved, allowing him to resume work and a "normal" life. It is impossible of course to estimate how many cases refractory to drug therapy also are due to abnormal GI motility, but it warrants consideration especially in the treatment of older patients with their notoriously unreliable bowel schedules.

Intestinal blood flow

One factor which we feel deserves more attention in any attempt to understand drug absorption in older subjects is the importance of blood flow to the intestinal area. Moreover, it is not only the intestinal perfusion relative to cardiac output which is important in any age-associated changes in drug absorption, but also the absolute change in such perfusion.

The effect of increasing age on the distribution of blood flow has been reviewed by Bender (1965b). Beyond age 20, the volume of blood pumped per unit time by the heart decreases at about 1% per year (Brandfonbrenner et al.,1955). This amounts to roughly a 30% decrease by age 65, but the distribution of blood is not reduced by a uniform 30% to each of the various body regions and tissues. Coronary circulation, for example, is largely unchanged and cerebral perfusion is down by only perhaps 14% by age 65. By contrast, blood flow to the liver, kidneys, and intestinal region is reduced by 40-50%.

Considering blood as the medium leeching drugs out of the intestine, one can easily imagine that reducing the rate (volume) of blood flow might reduce the drug concentration gradient across the serosal surface and slow the absorption of that drug. What information exists to assess the importance of this effect? For the most part, the studies on this point have involved administering drug solutions directly into the intestine of anesthetized animals, adjusting blood flow by means of an arterial clamp, and measuring either the amount of drug appearing in the blood or the amount remaining in the intestine. First-order kinetics were demonstrated in some cases (Diamond et al., 1970). Varro et al. (1965) found that sorbose absorption (by passive diffusion) was unaltered by decreasing blood flow to only 10% of the normal rate. Diamond et al. (1970) showed, however, that sulfaethidole absorption was very sensitive to decreases in circulation, dropping by 50% for a 35% reduction in flow. In addition, Haass et al. (1972) reported the rates of digoxin and digitoxin absorption to be perfusion-dependent (see figure 7). Winne and his colleagues studied the absorption of a variety of compounds and discovered that the absorption rate dependence is significant for some substances and decreases in the order: ethanol, methanol, glycerol, ethylene glycol, urea, erythritol, ribitol (Winne and Remischovsky, 1970). They noted that those compounds with the greatest dependence on blood flow were the ones with the greatest absorption rates and that the order of dependency paralleled the lipid solubility of the compounds (Winne, 1971). Ribitol absorption was totally independent of blood flow, as had been reported by Varro et al. (1965)for sorbose. Winne's group also found that, at neutral pH, antipyrine absorption and that of other basic compounds (amidopyrine, aniline) were directly correlated with blood flow (Ochsenfahrt and Winne, 1968a, 1968b, 1969). One of their curious observations stemmed from studies where the flow rate through the intestine was continuously varied and the absorption rate was likewise measured as a continuous function of flow rate. At intestinal pH values of 6 to 8, the basic compounds showed an increased absorption rate as the flow was increased and a decreased rate as the flow was decreased. Acidic compounds (salicylic acid, benzoic acid) were absorbed at a constant rate independent of increasing blood flow. Our interpretation is that a steady-state situation is approached for the absorption of compounds of high or moderate lipid solubility (sulfaethidole, digoxin, digitoxin, ethanol, methanol, etc. in the Winne and Remischovsky study (1970); and non-ionized basic compounds in the Ochsenfahrt and Winne studies (1968a, 1968b, 1969)), such that only as much compound is absorbed at the mucosal membrane as can be carried away from the serosal membrane by the blood. The dependency of absorption on blood flow rates is illustrated for a few drugs in figure 7. It might be pointed out that the steepness of the slopes in figure 7 is in the order of the compounds' lipid solubility. For compounds of low lipid solubility (sorbose, ribitol), it would appear that absorption at the mucosa is rate-limiting and that the blood flow will hardly affect this rate. The salicylic and benzoic acids, ionized at neutral pH, are at a disadvantage according to the pH-partition theory and probably do not satisfy the steady-state condition.

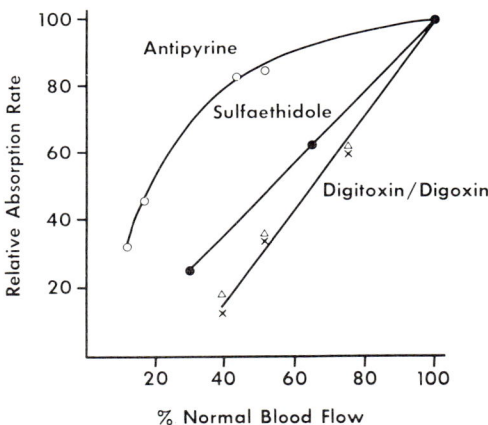

Fig. 7 Effect on intestinal drug absorption of varying blood flow. Data from Ochsenfahrt and Winne (1968a, b) for antipyrine; from Diamond et al. (1970) for sulfaethidole; and from Haass et al. (1972) for digitoxin and digoxin.

Blood flow rates also affect the absorption of glucose (Varro et al., 1965) and amino acids (Robinson et al., 1965), but these effects differ from those above in that these are active transport processes and the effect is mediated by metabolic effects, as mentioned earlier.

Obviously very little can be done to compensate for perfusion-related absorption defects of age. It may be of some utility however to remember that these particular defects occur primarily for highly potent lipophilic drugs, and this may be the unusual case where a larger dosage is required for the older patient.

Drug elimination

The peak drug level in the blood and the rate at which the blood level declines depends on the ability of the patient to metabolize and/or excrete the drug. Many human studies do not differentiate between metabolism and excretion however, but simply combine their effects in calculating the time required to reduce the blood level to one-half of a given value. This interval is called the half-life, or T/2, of drug elimination. Alternatively, an excretion or elimination constant (K_e) may be calculated according to pharmacokinetic models. Slow elimination of a drug is represented by a long T/2 or a small K_e.

Table III lists a few of the values for drug elimination in different age groups, and it is apparent that the overall elimination process is slower in older subjects. In some of the cases listed, it has been possible to distinguish whether the differences were due to altered metabolism or excretion, and these cases will be discussed below.

Metabolism

The operation of the kidney provides for the tubular reabsorption of lipid-soluble compounds from filtered plasma, thus effectively prolonging the action of many vitamins and drugs. Many such drugs are metabolized by enzymes in the liver -- the so-called hepatic microsomal hydroxylating system -- and converted to (multi) hydroxylated forms which may be 1) conjugated with glucuronic acid and excreted through the bile duct, 2) further oxidized and degraded, or 3) returned to the circulation and ultimately excreted by the kidney due to the more polar (less lipid-soluble) nature of the hydroxylated forms. This is of course primarily a detoxification mechanism built into the organism, but without it, our therapeutic cupboard would be decimated due to incidental drug toxicity. While drug metabolism is not solely the province of the liver, the contribution of other systems (kidney, plasma, GI mucosa) is relatively minor. A review of drug metabolism has been presented by Gorrod (1974).

In many cases, the duration of action of a drug is limited by the rate at which it is metabolized. There is evidence that drug metabolic patterns are altered in the older patient, and decreased detoxification capacity may be responsible for much of the adverse drug reaction liability

Table III

Drug Elimination in Old and Young Human Subjects

Drug	Subjects' Age	Plasma Half-life	K_e*	Reference
digoxin	27	51 hr	-	Ewy et al., 1969
	77	73 hr	-	
penicillin G	<50	males 23.7 min	-	Hansen et al., 1970
	>70	55.5 min	-	
	<30	females 20.7 min	-	Hansen et al., 1970
	>65	39.1 min	-	
antipyrine	26	12.0 hr	-	O'Malley et al., 1971
	78	17.4 hr	-	
phenylbuta-zone	26	81.2 hr	-	O'Malley et al., 1971
	78	104.6 hr	-	
dihydro-streptomycin	25	5.2 hr	-	Vartia and Leikola, 1960
	76	8.4 hr	-	
aminopyrine	25-30	3 hr	-	Jori et al., 1972
	65-85	10 hr	-	
diazepam	17-59	-	.30	Garattini et al., 1973
	60-80	-	.15	
xylose	30-49	-	.40	Guth, 1968
	80+	-	.08	

*Calculated from the investigators' data as fitted to a one-compartment model. We are grateful to Dr. W. Westlake of Smith, Kline & French Laboratories for these calculations.

of this patient group. The seminal work in this area is that of Streicher and Garbus (1955) who were studying the duration of sleep induced in rats by hexobarbital. They found that rats of both sexes showed age-related changes in susceptibility and that these changes were related to the development and decline in sex hormone levels in both sexes. Kato et al. (1964, 1970a, 1970c) extended these observations to the metabolism and pharmacological response for several drugs in rats of different ages. Figure 8 shows that there is good correlation of the hepatic microsomal metabolism of a drug, its serum level, and the response to the drug. At least for animals of sexual maturity or older, the rate of drug metabolism apparently limits the extent of the pharmacologic response by regulating the level of the circulating drug.

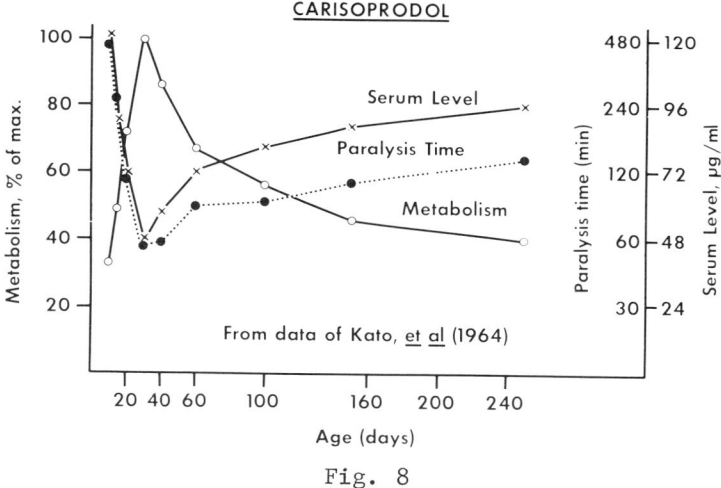

Fig. 8

These relationships are expressed in a different manner in figure 9, which also shows that the total carisoprodol metabolism by the body is probably due to the liver. It was furthermore noted by the Kato group that -- for some drugs -- animals of different ages appear to have the same responsiveness to a given blood concentration and that differences in these animals' response to an equal oral dose were due to differences in metabolic clearance of the drug. This view is supported by the work of Kuhlmann et al. (1970) who found that the longer sleep time of older rats is not due to an altered ED_{50} for the anesthetic. They showed furthermore that hexobarbital is metabolized more slowly by older rats, but that barbital (which is not metabolized at all) gives rise to equal sleep times for older and younger rats.

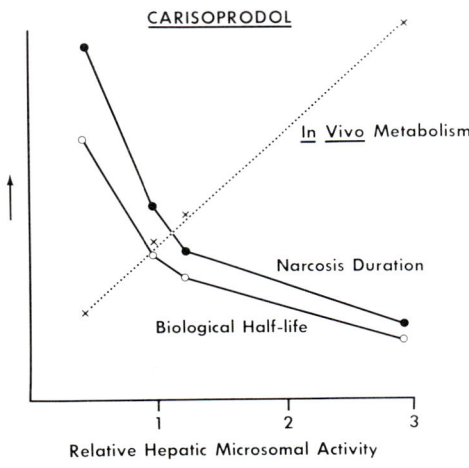

Fig. 9

A number of human studies of age-dependent drug metabolism have been reported. One group of subjects, average age 75, exhibited a metabolic half-life for aminopyrine of about twice that observed for a group under age 30 (Jori et al., 1972). (This same age-related difference was reported for rats (Klinger, 1969) and, like Kato's studies, was reflected by similar differences in drug metabolism by liver microsomes from different aged animals.) O'Malley et al. (1971) found a slightly smaller increase (45%) for antipyrine plasma half-life in an elderly group, and reported also a 29% decrease in phenylbutazone metabolism. Phenylbutazone, it will be recalled, is fairly toxic in general and especially so in older patients, probably largely due to impaired metabolic detoxification. Another prominent adverse drug reaction of the elderly is their special sensitivity to barbiturates, resulting in confusion and CNS depression. This reaction is very likely due to reduced metabolism, as it is found that older subjects show only half the rate of amylobarbitone hydroxylation shown by younger ones (Irvine et al., 1974). Higher plasma levels of amylobarbitone were also established in the older people.

The view that many of the adverse drug reactions suffered by older patients are due to a declining capacity for drug metabolism is simple and appealing. Presumably a situation arises where the daily drug intake is not balanced by the metabolism of that drug to a less active or more readily excreted form. The unusually high level of active drug may then give rise to an excessive primary pharmacological response or to a greater expression of secondary side effects. This situation is only more aggravated by the great drug load placed on the metabolic system by the multiple drug burden common to these patients. An example of this was cited earlier and demonstrated the impact of only one additional drug on another's metabolism; consider the magnitude of this effect in a patient taking several drugs. The greater incidence of ADR in elderly women (relative to elderly men) probably also derives from metabolic factors, as older women show slower antipyrine metabolism (O'Malley et al., 1971) and maintain higher serum aminopyrine levels (Jori et al., 1974) than older males. It has proved difficult however to define the biochemical processes and interactions responsible for this phenomenon of age- and sex-related hepatic metabolism changes, due to species differences among the animals employed in relevant studies (Kato et al., 1970a, b, c, d). The most commonly espoused explanations invoke some involvement of androgens and estrogens with hepatic regulatory processes, but additional species factors must be involved. Whatever these factors, all the species and strains studied show an inverse relationship of drug metabolism rate and pharmacologic effect.

While it is useful to recognize that the (drug) metabolic capacity diminishes with age (and especially so for women) and that this may lead to prolonged drug action or toxic drug reactions, it is nevertheless difficult to anticipate its importance accurately. For one thing, there is an enormous individual variability in drug metabolism, apparently genetically inherited (Vesell and Page, 1968a,b). Furthermore, since there are actually multiple metabolic pathways existing for drugs, a patient's metabolic capacity for antipyrine will not help estimate his phenylbutazone metabolic rate. There is even some suggestion that physical activity directly affects metabolism of drugs (Levy, 1967) although this has not been explored well enough to be characterized. Finally, the administration of drugs which induce or inhibit hepatic hydroxylating enzymes is of obvious importance, as described under Drug Interactions, and, in addition to affecting its own metabolism or that of other drugs, can interfere with normal body metabolism to give rise to idiopathic ailments.

Excretion

As noted in the preceding section, drugs of high lipid solubility are cleared from the body by conversion to more polar forms which are excreted along with other body wastes as well as with drugs of intrinsically poor lipid solubility. If metabolic conversion is often the rate-limiting step in clearing the highly lipid soluble drug, renal excretion itself is rate-limiting for clearance of the others and sometimes for drug metabolite clearance also. This clearance occurs for most polar compounds simply by glomerular filtration, since they are not well reabsorbed in the renal tubule. Organic acids however may be actively excreted at the tubule by specific transport systems, as is the case for penicillin metabolites. Certain drugs are secreted in the bile as mentioned earlier, but these are few relative to those cleared by the kidney.

It is useful in considering renal function to return to the information presented earlier about blood flow redistribution with age. Blood flow to the kidneys and liver was estimated to drop by about 1.5% per year after maturity, so that it is roughly 40-45% lower at age 65 than at 25. The effect of this decrease on drug clearance characteristics is roughly comparable to the blood flow decrement, with both glomerular filtration rate (GFR) and urea clearance down by 45% (Holloway, 1974) and blood urea nitrogen (BUN) accordingly up by 50% (Lewis and Irving, 1953). An additional 10-20% decrease in GFR may occur as a result of β-block therapy (Ibsen and Sederberg-Olsen, 1973), and, while this may be of little importance for young patients, it may precipitate a serious drug clearance problem for the aged. It is not useful to use serum creatinine levels as an index of renal function, since they do not show a drop until creatinine clearance has decreased by about 50% (Hansen et al., 1970) the serum level being maintained constant up to that point by decreased creatinine synthesis. Let us review briefly the effects of altered excretory function on drug handling by older patients.

The retention of bromsulphalein (BSP) is a common test for liver function. It has been reported (Thompson and Williams, 1965) that retention of BSP by subjects over the age of 70 was double that of those under 40, indicating a progressive loss of liver function, and this was attributed to a comparable fall in liver storage capacity. DeLeeuw-Israel et al. (1969) also found the storage capacity to be decreased, but reported maximal biliary excretion and removal of BSP from circulation to be little altered in older subjects. Other studies (Calloway and Merrill, 1965; Koff et al., 1973) tend to bear out this latter view that there is no significant age-related change in liver function with regard to drug clearance.

Contrary to the situation with respect to liver, the kidneys' effectiveness in drug clearance is significantly reduced in older subjects. Renal function correlates well with the ADR incidence (Smith et al., 1966), in fact, and is probably the reason for the greatest amount of ADR in elderly patients. Digoxin administered intravenously to elderly men reached serum levels twice that achieved by younger men (Ewy et al., 1969), probably due to renal differences since digoxin clearance was 53 ml/min for the older and 83 ml/min for the younger men. A similar dependency of clearance volumes on age was noted for xylose and inulin (Guth, 1968).

A large number of examples of antibiotic half-life dependence on age have been reported and show clearly that renal tubular secretion is impaired essentially in parallel with the decrease in renal blood flow. Vartia and Leikola (1960) found that i.m.-administered penicillin-G was resorbed equally well in adult human subjects of all ages. However, penicillin-G, as well as dihydrostreptomycin, procaine penicillin, and tetracycline (Leikola and Vartia, 1957) all reached much higher average levels in elderly patients than in young ones and the rate of serum level decrease was also slower (see also figure 10). Although penicillin V is absorbed relatively slowly from the intestines of aged rats, these same rats had higher serum levels of the drug than did younger rats with much more rapid absorption (Niedermuller et al., 1974). Hansen et al. (1970) and Gingell and Waterworth (1968) showed that creatinine clearance is a good index of antibiotic clearance. The dependence of antibiotic clearance on renal blood flow (as represented by creatinine clearance) is illustrated for several different examples in figure 11 (Hitzenberger, 1971). This relationship holds for digoxin as well (Ewy et al., 1969).

Considering that virtually all older people possess significantly reduced renal function, we must expect that they will achieve serum drug levels roughly twice that anticipated for that same dosage administered to a younger adult. This level of course may be much more than twice normal if the patient also has a reduced drug metabolizing capacity, which means that the risk of adverse drug reaction is proportionately increased.

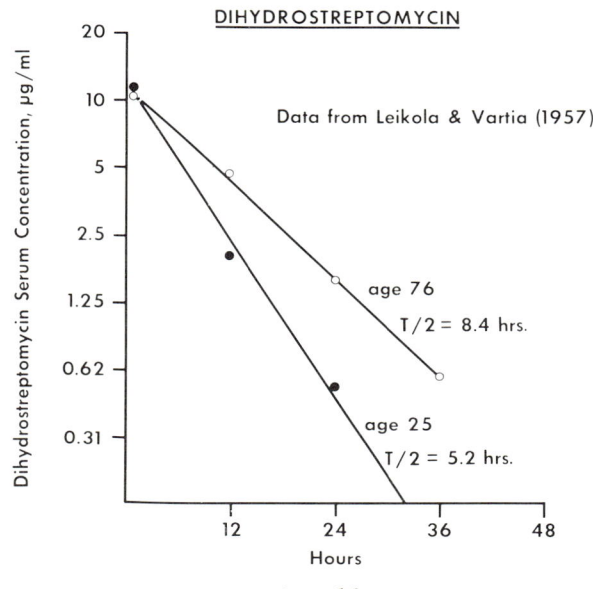

Fig. 10

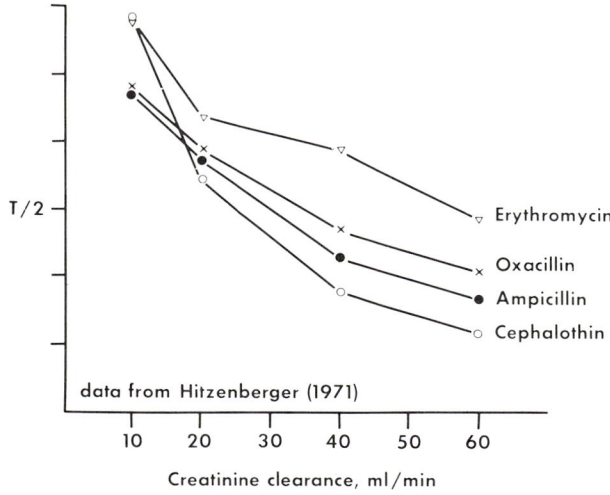

Fig. 11

SUMMARY

We have reviewed the effect of age on the absorption, metabolism, and excretion of drugs. This subject is of practical interest because these changes lead to abnormal drug levels in the circulation and, consequently, to an increased risk of adverse/toxic reactions or inadequate therapeutic response. Drug absorption is apparently reduced in many cases, a combined result of retarded GI motility and decreased GI blood flow, and may lead to an ineffective serum drug level. By far the more important change with age, and the best documented, is a reduction in the rate at which drugs are metabolized and eliminated. This affords a prolonged drug action, but is accompanied by the potential for excessive physiological response or other adverse drug effects. Nevertheless, with some consideration for all these age-related changes, it is possible to anticipate the types of problems each prescription may present for the older patient and to be prepared accordingly to institute appropriate changes in dosage or therapeutic agent.

REFERENCES

Archambault, R. F. (1974). J. Am. Med. Assoc. 230, 960.
Ayd, J. F. (1961). J. Am. Med. Assoc. 175, 1054.
Baron, J. H. (1963). Gut 4, 136.
Bender, A. D. (1965a). Exp. Gerontol. 1, 237.
Bender, A. D. (1965b). J. Am. Geriat. Soc. 13, 192.
Bender, A. D. (1968). J. Am. Geriat. Soc. 16, 1331.
Bender, A. D. (1974). J. Am. Geriat. Soc. 22, 296.
Bianchine, J. R., Calimlim, L. R., Morgan, J. P., Dujuvne, C. A., and Lasagna, L. (1971). Ann. N.Y. Acad. Sci. 179, 126.
Brandfonbrenner, M., Landowne, M., and Shock, N. W. (1955). Circulation 12, 557.
Briganti, F. J. (1973). In "Drugs and the Elderly" (R. H. Davis and W. K. Smith, eds.), pp. 25-32, Ethel Percy Andrus Gerontology Center, Los Angeles.
Calloway, N. O., and Merrill, R. S. (1965). J. Am. Geriat. Soc. 13, 594.
Caranasos, G. J., Stewart, R. B., and Cluff, L. E. (1974). J. Am. Med. Assoc. 228, 713.
Cluff, L. E. (1967). Hospital Practice 2, 101.
Davis, R. K., Tucker, G. J., and Harrow, M. (1971). Am. J. Psychiat. 128, 95.
Davis, R. L., Lawton, A. H., Prouty, R., and Chow, B. F. (1965). J. Gerontol. 20, 169.

DeBosset, P. L., and Bitter, T. (1973). *Schweiz. Med. Wochschr.* 103, 1153.
deLeeuw-Israel, F. R., Hollander, C. F., and Arp-Neefjes, J. M. (1969). *J. Gerontol.* 24, 140.
Diamond, L., Doluisio, J. T., and Crouthamel, W. G. (1970). *European J. Pharmacol.* 11, 109.
Dietze, V. F., Kalbe, I., Kranz, D., Bruschke, G., and Richter, H. (1971). *Z. Alternsforsch.* 24, 229.
Draper, H. H. (1958). *Proc. Soc. Exp. Biol. Med.* 97, 121.
Ewy, G. A., Kapadia, G. G., Yao, L., Lullin, M., and Marcus, F. I. (1969). *Circulation* 39, 449.
Fann, W. E. (1973). *Southern Med. J.* 66, 661.
Field, J. B., Ohta, M., Boyle, C., and Remer, A. (1967). *New Engl. J. Med.* 277, 889.
Fikry, M. E., and Aboul-Wafa, M. H. (1965). *Gerontol. Clin.* 7, 171.
Freeman, J. T. (1965). "Clinical Features of the Older Patient". Charles C Thomas, Springfield, Illinois.
Furcht, L. T., and Scott, R. E. (1973). *J. Cell. Biol.* 59, 106a.
Garattini, S., Marcucci, F., Morselli, P. L., and Mussini, E. (1973). In "Biological Effects of Drugs in Relation to their Plasma Concentrations" (D. S. Davies and B. N. C. Prichard, eds.), pp. 211-225, University Park Press, Baltimore.
Gingell, J. C., and Waterworth, P. M. (1968). *Brit. Med. J.* 2, 19.
Gorrod, J. W. (1974). *Gerontol. Clin.* 16, 30.
Guth, P. H. (1968). *Am. J. Digest. Diseases* 13, 565.
Gwilt, J. R., Robertson, A., Goldman, L., and Blanchard, A. W. (1963). *J. Pharm. Pharmacol.* 15, 445.
Haass, A., Lullmann, H., and Peters, T. (1972). *European J. Pharmacol.* 19, 366.
Hall, M. R. P. (1973). *Brit. Med. J.* 3, 582.
Hansch, C., and Fujita, T. (1964). *J. Am. Chem. Soc.* 86, 1616.
Hansen, J. M., Kampmann, J., and Laursen, H. (1970). *Lancet* i, 1170.
Heading, R. C., Nimmo, J., Prescott, L. F., and Tothill, P. (1973). *Brit. J. Pharmacol.* 47, 415.
Hitzenberger, G. (1971). *Deut. Med. Wochschr.* 96, 1805.
Hoddinott, B. C., Gowdey, C. W., Coulter, W. K., and Parker, J. M. (1967). *Can. Med. Assoc. J.* 97, 1001.
Holloway, D. A. (1974). *Drug Intell. Clin. Pharmacol.* 8, 632.
Hurwitz, N. (1969). *Brit. Med. J.* 1, 536.
Hyams, D. E. (1964). *Gerontol. Clin.* 6, 193.

Ibsen, H., and Sederberg-Olsen, P. (1973). Clin. Med. 44, 129.
Irvine, R. E., Grove, J., Toseland, P. A., and Trounce, J. R. (1974). Brit. J. Clin. Pharmacol. 1, 41.
Jacobs, A. M., and Owens, G. M. (1969). J. Gerontol. 24, 95.
Janowsky, D. S., Davis, J. M., and El-Yousef, M. K. (1974). In "Drug Issues in Geropsychiatry" (W. E. Fann and G. L. Maddox, eds.), pp. 19-28, Williams & Wilkins, Baltimore.
Jones, T. (1962). J. Am. Geriat. Soc. 10, 259.
Jori, A., DiSalle, E., and Quadri, A. (1972). Pharmacology 8, 273.
Kato, R., and Takanaka, A. (1968). Japan. J. Pharmacol. 18, 389.
Kato, R., Vassanelli, P., Frontino, K., and Chiesara, E. (1964). Biochem. Pharmacol. 13, 1037.
Kato, R., Onoda, K-I., and Takanaka, A. (1970a). Japan. J. Pharmacol. 20, 546.
Kato, R., Onoda, K-I., and Takanaka, A. (1970b). Japan. J. Pharmacol. 20, 554.
Kato, R., Onoda, K-I., and Takanaka, A. (1970c). Japan. J. Pharmacol. 20, 562.
Kato, R., Takanaka, A., and Onoda, K-I. (1970d). Japan. J. Pharmacol. 20, 572.
Kekki, M., Pyorala, K., Mustala, O., Salmi, H., Jussila, J., and Siurala, M. (1971). Intern. J. Clin. Pharmacol. 2, 209.
Klinger, W. (1969). Arch. Intern. Pharmacodyn. 180, 309.
Koff, R. S., Garvey, A. J., Burney, S. W., and Bell, B. (1973). Gastroenterology 65, 300.
Kojima, S., Smith, R. B., and Doluisio, J. T. (1971). J. Pharm. Sci. 60, 1639.
Kuhlmann, K., Oduah, M., and Coper, H. (1970). Naunyn-Schmiedebergs Arch. Exp. Pathol. Pharmakol. 265, 310.
Lamy, P. P. (1974). Clin. Med. 81, 52.
Lamy, P. P., and Kitler, M. E. (1971). J. Am. Geriat. Soc. 19, 23.
Lee, P. V. (1972). Med. World News, Geriatrics Issue, p. 27.
Leikola, E., and Vartia, K. O. (1957). J. Gerontol. 12, 48.
Levine, R. R. (1970). Am. J. Digest. Diseases 15, 171.
Levy, G. (1967). J. Pharm. Sci. 56, 928.
Lewis, W., and Irving, A. S. (1953). Am. J. Physiol. 8, 446.
Linn, B. S. (1975). This Symposium.
Lipscomb, H. S., Muecke, A. H., and Stevens, D. (1973). Med. World News, Geriatrics Issue, pp. 32-38.
Marcus, C. S., and Lengemann, F. W. (1962). J. Nutr. 77, 155.
Meldrum, S. J., Watson, B. W., and Riddle, H. C. (1972). Brit. Med. J. 2, 104.

Modell, W. (guest ed.) (1974). *Geriatrics* **29**, 50.
Morselli, P. L., Garattini, S., and Cohen, S. N. (eds.)(1974). "Drug Interactions". Raven Press, New York.
Niedermuller, H., Hofecker, G., and Kment, A. (1974). *Experientia* **30**, 214.
Nies, A. S. (1974). *Med. Clin. No. Am.* **58**, 965.
Nimmo, J., Heading, R. C., and Prescott, L. F. (1971). *Scot. Med. J.* **16**, 337.
Ochsenfahrt, H., and Winne, D. (1968a). *Life Sci.* **7** (I), 493.
Ochsenfahrt, H., and Winne, D. (1968b). *Naunyn-Schmiedebergs Arch. Exp. Pathol. Pharmakol.* **260**, 184.
Ochsenfahrt, H., and Winne, D. (1969). *Naunyn-Schmiedebergs Arch. Exp. Pathol. Pharmakol.* **264**, 55.
O'Malley, K., Crooks, J., Duke, E., and Stevenson, I. H. (1971). *Brit. Med. J.* **3**, 607.
Pelz, K. S., Gottfried, S. P., and Soos, E. (1968). *Geriatrics* **23**, 149.
Pemberton, M. (1954). *Brit. Med. J.* **1**, 490.
Penzes, L. (1970). *Exp. Gerontol.* **5**, 193.
Penzes, L. (1974). *Exp. Gerontol.* **9**, 245, 253, 259.
Penzes, L., Simon, G., and Winter, M. (1968). *Exp. Gerontol.* **3**, 321.
Pottage, A., Nimmo, J., and Prescott, L. F. (1974). *J. Pharm. Pharmacol.* **26**, 144.
Prescott, L. F. (1974a). *Brit. J. Clin. Pharmacol.* **1**, 189.
Prescott, L. F. (1974b). *Med. Clin. No. Am.* **58**, 907.
Redl, G., Cramer, R. D., and Berkoff, C. E. (1974). *Chem. Soc. Rev.* **3**, 273.
Rivera-Calimlim, L., Morgan, J. P., Dujuvne, C. A., Bianchine, J. R., and Lasagna, L. (1970). *Clin. Res.* **18**, 343.
Robinson, J. W. L., Jequier, J-C., Felber, J. P., and Mirkovitch, V. (1965). *J. Surg. Res.* **5**, 150.
Rowland, M., Matin, S. B., Thiessen, J., and Karam, J. (1974). *In* "Drug Interactions" (P. L. Morselli, S. Garattini, and S. N. Cohen, eds.), pp. 199-210, Raven Press, New York.
Sapp, O. L., Seasions, J. T., and Rose, J. W. (1964). *Clin. Res.* **12**, 31.
Schachter, D., Dowdle, E. B., and Schenker, H. (1960). *Am. J. Physiol.* **198**, 263, 275.
Seidl, L. G., Thornton, G. F., Smith, J. W., and Cluff, L. E. (1966). *Bull. Johns Hopkins Hosp.* **119**, 299.
Sheppard, J. R. (1972). *Nature New Biol.* **236**, 14.
Shock, N. W. (1961). *Ann. Rev. Physiol.* **23**, 97.

Siurala, M., Mustala, O., and Jussila, J. (1969). Scand. J. Gastroenterol. 4, 269.
Smith, J. W., Seidl, L. G., and Cluff, L. E. (1966). Ann. Internal Med. 65, 629.
Sotaniemi, E. A. (1973). Pharmacology 10, 306.
Sotaniemi, E. A., and Palva, I. P. (1972). Ann. Clin. Res. 4, 158.
Sotaniemi, E. A., Ylostalo, P. R., and Kauppila, A. J. (1974). European J. Clin. Pharmacol. 7, 473.
Streicher, E., and Garbus, J. (1955). J. Gerontol. 10, 441.
Task Force on Prescription Drugs, Final Report (1969). p. 2, U. S. Dept. HEW, Washington, D. C.
Thompson, E. N., and Williams, R. (1965). Gut 6, 266.
Varro, V., Blaho, G., Csernay, L., Jung, I., and Szarvas, F. (1965). Am. J. Digest Diseases 10, 170.
Vartia, K. O., and Leikola, E. (1960). J. Gerontol. 15, 392.
Vesell, E. S., and Page, J. G. (1968a). Science 159, 1479.
Vesell, E. S., and Page, J. G. (1968b). Science 161, 72.
Wasserman, R. H., and Taylor, A. N. (1968). J. Biol. Chem. 243, 3987.
Weg. R. (1973). In "Drugs and the Elderly" (R. H. Davis and W. K. Smith, eds.), pp. 71-91, Ethel Percy Andrus Gerontology Center, Los Angeles.
Wilson, J. P. (1967). Gut 8, 618.
Wilson, L. A., Lawson, I. R., and Brass, W. (1962). Lancet ii, 7261.
Winne, D. (1971). Med. Welt 22, 632.
Winne, D., and Remischovsky, J. (1970). J. Pharm. Pharmacol. 22, 640.
Witton, K., and Herrman, H. T. (1963). Diseases Nervous System 24, 314.
Yeh, S. D. J., Soltz, W., and Chow, B. F. (1965). J. Gerontol. 20, 177.

BIOPHYSICAL ASPECTS OF RED CELL AGING

David Danon

Section of Biological Ultrastructure
The Weizmann Institute of Science
Rehovot, Israel

The death of a cell may be considered as a progressive phenomenon, a kind of telescoped death of a higher organism in miniature (Bessis, 1964). The senescence of a cell may be considered similarly. Investigations of the mechanism and characteristics of cellular aging represent, therefore, a larger scope than the aging of a minute part of an organ of the body. The choice of a model for such a study may be directed either by consideration of the importance of the cell to be investigated, or by its relative simplicity in terms of anatomy, biochemistry and physiology, and, therefore, the probability that it offers to elucidate some basic problems in the process of cellular aging.

From this point of view, the mammalian red blood cell is a very suitable model for the study of aging at the cellular level.

After the initial differentiation to the erythroid line, every cell division is followed by changes leading to the final specialization, i.e., to the erythrocyte. After three or four cell divisions, the nucleus is expelled (Skutelsky and Danon, 1967). The remaining reticulocyte which enters the circulation contains some polyribosomes and monosomes, mRNA, t-RNA and essential enzymes for protein synthesis (Lowenstein, 1959; Marks et al., 1963) as well as some mitochondria and other membraneous organelles. During the process of maturation, the reticulocyte loses all its intracellular organelles. Its capacity for protein synthesis gradually decreases until finally no protein synthesis takes place. The mature erythrocyte contains no mitochondria and consumes only minute amounts of oxygen through the pentose shunt (Schweiger, 1962). The existence of mitochondria and the high rate of oxygen consumption by reticulocytes was considered to be the explanation for the high content of ATP in reticulocytes (Brok et al., 1966). It was later proved that a functional tricarboxylic acid cycle exists in reticulocytes (Gasko and Danon, 1972a) and that a decline in this metabolic pathway is associated with reticulocyte maturation (Gasko and Danon, 1972b). During this final stage of maturation of the reticulocyte, the mitochondria and other membraneous organelles are expelled or disintegrated intracellularly (Kent et al., 1966; Gasko and Danon, 1972b). The remodeling of the membrane takes place by endocytosis and by exocytosis (Gasko and Danon, 1974). During this last stage of maturation, the surface charge density of the reticulocyte is slightly increased (Stephens, 1940; Walter et al., 1965; Skutelsky and Danon, 1970).

GENERAL CHANGES WITH AGE

The mature erythrocyte is a bidiscoidal cell composed of a cell membrane which contains its full complement of hemoglobin and a variety of enzymes. These enzymes catalyze the reactions required for its physiological function and the maintenance of its structure. The cell is, however, no longer capable of new synthesis of enzymes or other proteins. The cell has all its structural and functional components but no capacity for renewal by resynthesis. Therefore, the erythrocyte, once in the circulation, will have its survival time determined by whatever mechanism except the incapacity to reproduce enzymes or membranes. Errors in protein structure are also excluded. In other words, the aging of the erythrocyte is a one-way traffic.

For many years, the research on the aging of the mammalian erythrocyte was focused on the capacity of this cell to provide the energy necessary for its function. A considerable amount of work was devoted to the levels of enzymatic activity inside these cells as a function of their age (Marks, 1961; Pennel, 1964; Brok et al., 1966).

In 1966, we drew attention to the fact that hemolysis in the circulation is a rare occurrence under physiological conditions. Senescent cells that reach their term are normally sequestrated in the reticulo-endothelial system (Danon, 1966). The question was raised whether the structural alterations evidenced by biophysical methods precede, or follow, enzymatic insufficiency in the aging erythrocyte.

The fact that no enzyme of major importance is diminished in its activity to less than half the activity of the whole population of cells and even ATP levels are not lower than half the average level (Marks, 1961; Pennel, 1964; Brok et al., 1966), has shifted our interest to a new question: What is it that the macrophage recognizes in the old erythrocyte so as to identify it as an "undesirable self" or as a "deteriorated self"?

The information accumulated during the years on the biophysical parameters that change with the age of the erythrocyte may be summarized as follows: As the red cell ages, its diameter decreases, its osmotic resistance decreases and so does its capacity to change its form in narrow passages and recover it. In terms of a laboratory test, we may say that its reversible deformability or its mechanical resistance decrease. The granularity on the surface of the red cell membrane as visualized by electron microscopy is diminished and, similarly, there is a diminution of the stromalytic forms obtained by the negative staining technique (Danon, 1966).

The mobility of the cells in an electric field (electrophoresis) was found to be slower in the old erythrocyte (Danon and Marikovsky, 1961; Yaari, 1969). Similar information on the reduction in surface charge density was reported by Walter et al. in 1965 using the counter current distribution method for separating erythrocytes. The surface charge density was found to be diminished in old erythrocytes by another indirect method. Using the Fragiligraph with an accessory for automatic recording of agglutinability (Danon et al., 1969), we have shown that old erythrocytes are agglutinated by poly-L-lysine at a higher rate and reach a higher plateau than young ones, indicating a lower repulsion force between the cells. Agglutinability by antibodies showed a similar difference between old and young cells. Old red blood cells were found to have higher resistance to acid fragility (Danon, 1966) and higher immune lysis (Danon, 1966).

CHANGES IN SURFACE CHARGE DENSITY

When all these parameters are reviewed and examined as to the probability of each of them to serve as a recognition sign for the sequestration in the spleen, two properties of the old red blood cell were primarily suspect, viz., the reduction in reversible deformability and the reduction in surface charge density. Since the reduction in reversible deformability was found to be associated with the reduction in ATP levels, several authors have considered this parameter to be of primary importance in determining the survival of the erythrocytes in the circulation (Burton, 1970; Weed et al., 1969). However, experiments carried out in our laboratory in 1971 (Elazar et al., 1971) showed that about 80% of young rabbit erythrocytes, treated with neuraminidase so as to lose about half their sialic acid, were removed from the circulation within 16 hours (figure 1). These cells were unaltered as far as their osmotic fragility, their reversible deformability, their ATP levels and their G6PD levels. We have thus considered the sialic acid negative charge density on the surface of erythrocytes, that is remarkably diminished on the old red blood cells and on the surface of neuraminidase-treated cells, as a most probable sign of recognition by the macrophage. Studies from another laboratory have similarly shown that red cells treated with neuraminidase and with trypsin and reinjected into the circulation left the circulation within a few hours (Halbhuber et al., 1972). These results, as well as our own on the neuraminidase-treated cells, could be criticized. It was difficult to exclude the possibility that some molecules of neuraminidase remained attached to the surface of the cells that were reinjected into the host animal after labeling with chromium. Therefore, the cells may have been identified by the macrophages, not only as deteriorated self cells but also as cells coated with "non-self" molecules of neuraminidase and, therefore, phagocytized as "non-self".

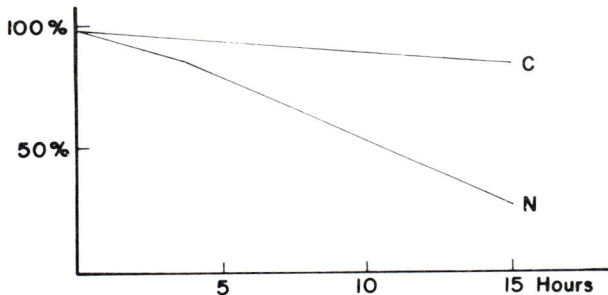

Fig. 1 Rabbit erythrocytes treated with neuraminidase (N) and controls (C) reinjected into rabbits after labeling with radiochromium. Note the rapid disappearance of the neuraminidase-treated cells.

We needed another example of a cellular element that is "recognized" by the macrophage and phagocytized, to be excluded, as a "deteriorated self". At that time, we knew already (Skutelsky and Danon, 1967) that the nucleus of the late erythroblast is extruded from the cell in a manner similar to a mitotic division so as to result, on the one hand, in the future reticulocyte and in a nucleus surrounded by a narrow rim of cytoplasm and cell membrane, on the other (figure 2). Here we had another example of a cell membrane that is a "self" and is recognized by the macrophage as "undesirable self" and phagocytized. It was impossible to isolate free nuclei and submit them to electrophoresis. We have, therefore, adopted the method described by Gassic et al. in 1968 using colloidal iron as cell surface electron stain. With this method, we first tried to evaluate the charge density by counting the number of colloidal iron particles on the surface of cells, on electron micrographs and comparing them with the data obtained by electrophoresis (Marikovsky and Danon, 1969). The agreement between the two methods was satisfactory except for the fact that no iron particles were found in the cells treated with neuraminidase, while cells similarly treated did migrate in the electric field to about 15% of the velocity of the young cells. However, we were satisfied with the fact that old cells migrated slower than young ones by about 30% and that was also approximately the lower proportion of iron particles counted in the micrographs of old cells as compared with young cells (figure 3).

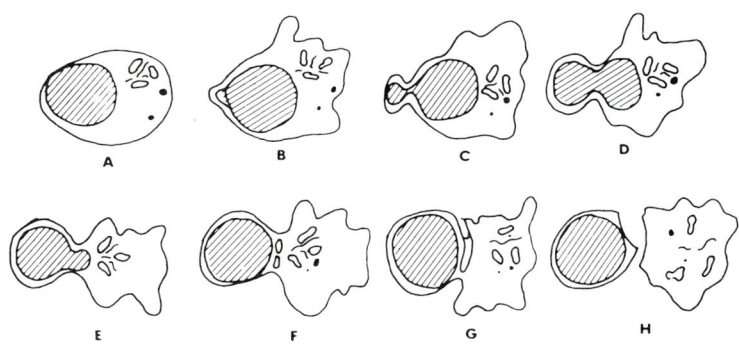

Fig. 2 A schematic representation of the expulsion of the nucleus from the late erythroblast of a rabbit. The nucleus first occupies an excentric position (A). It is then gradually extruded (B,C,D,E). Vacuole-like separation takes place (F), and the vacuoles enlarge until a single filament keeps the continuity between the extruded nucleus and the future reticulocyte (G). When this is interrupted, the nucleus, surrounded by a narrow rim of cytoplasm and cell membrane (H), will be separated from the reticulocyte (Skutelsky and Danon, 1967).

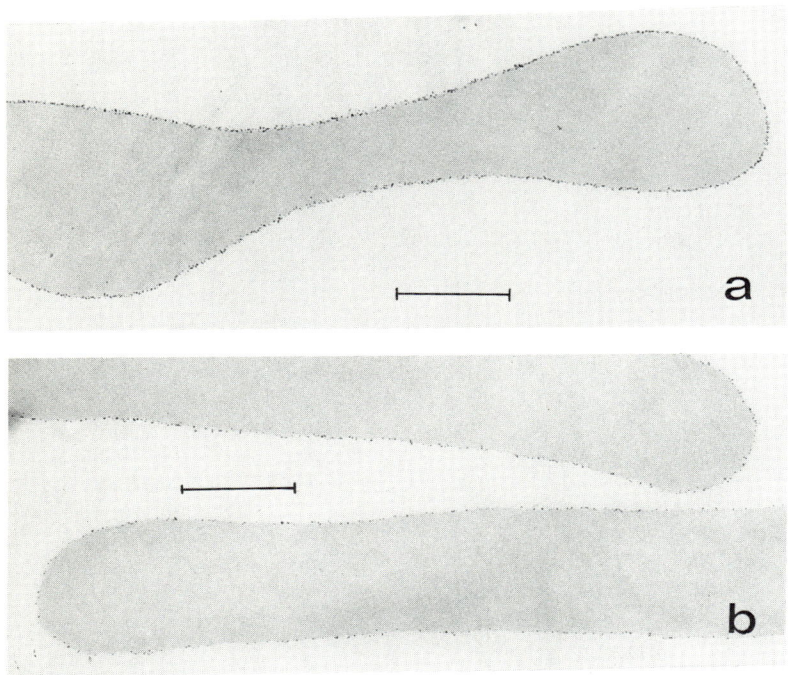

Fig. 3 Young (A) and old (B) human red blood cells labeled with colloidal iron (Gassic et al., 1968) for evaluation of their surface charge density. Note the lesser density of the colloidal iron particles on the old cells (B). Magnification X25,000. (Marikovsky and Danon, 1969.)

Using the same method for labeling, we were now able to evaluate the surface charge density on the membrane of the expelled nucleus. As a matter of fact, we have found (Skutelsky and Danon, 1969) that even before the nucleus is completely expelled there is already a marked difference in charge density between the membrane that will surround the remaining reticulocyte and the one that bulges out with the nucleus that will be extruded (figure 4). The extruded nucleus therefore had lesser charge density than the remaining reticulocyte and was probably identified by the macrophage as a candidate for phagocytosis. In an analysis of the surface charge labeling density at various stages of the erythroid line (Skutelsky and Danon, 1970), the results indicated that the biosynthesis of n-acetyl neuraminic acid stops at the earliest recognizable stage of erythroid differentiation and, therefore, the charge density is diminished after each cell division (figure 5).

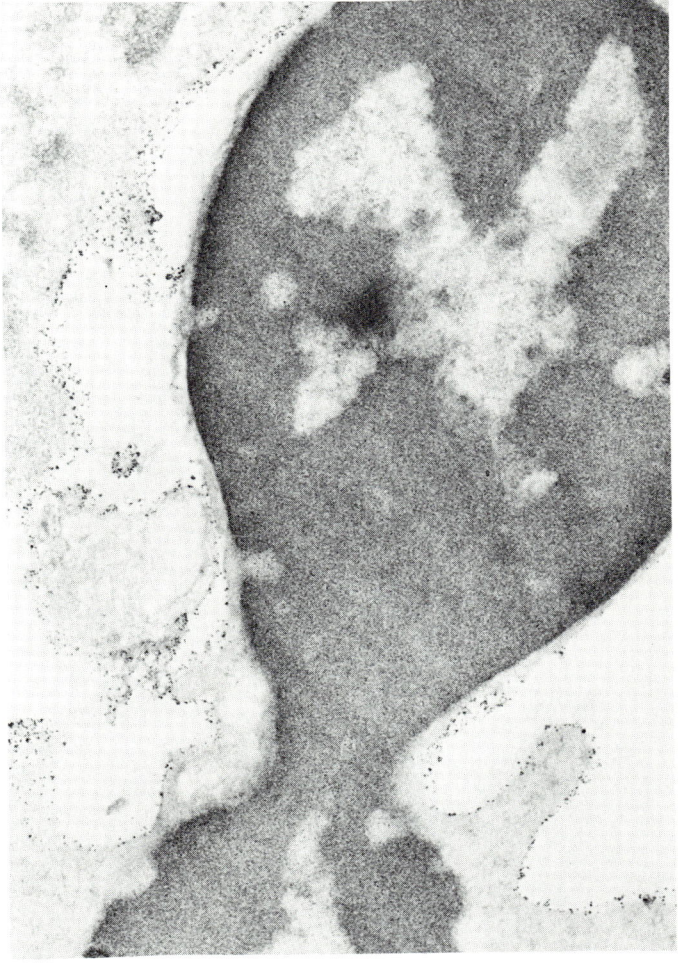

Fig. 4 An erythroid nucleus in the process of being extruded from an erythroblast in the bone marrow of a rabbit, labeled with colloidal iron for evaluation of surface charge density. Note the lower density of particles on the membrane that surrounds the extruded part of the nucleus as compared with the part that remains to become a reticulocyte. This is particularly well seen on the lower right. An erythroblast at early stage of differentiation with higher charge density is seen on top left (Skutelsky and Danon, 1970).

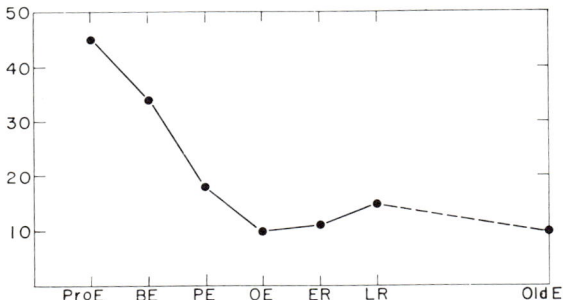

Fig. 5 Charge density on the surface of erythroid cells as a function of their degree of differentiation. On the ordinate, the number of particles in a unit length of perpendicularly sectioned cell membrane in the bone marrow of a rabbit labeled with colloidal iron. On the abcissa, the degree of differentiation. Pro E - ProErythroblast. BE - Basophilic Erythroblast. PE - Polychromatic Erythroblast. OE - Orthochromatic Erythroblast. ER - Early Reticulocyte. LR - Late Reticulocyte. Old E - Old Erythrocyte. (Skutelsky and Danon, 1970.)

Last year, Jancik and Schauer (1974) published a paper in which they proved that rabbit erythrocytes are not able to regenerate their membrane sialic acids, concluding that exogenous factors such as serum neuraminidase may have great influence upon the lifetime of erythrocytes. In addition, last year Gattegno et al. (1974) reported that neuraminidase-treated and intact rabbit erythrocytes have similar in vitro properties, except those of cellular charge and cellular adhesion, in their sera. However, after injection into rabbits, the sialic acid-free erythrocytes were promptly removed from circulation, whereas intact erythrocytes, previously incubated under the same conditions but without neuraminidase, were removed from circulation after a significantly longer period.

Surface negative charge did not seem to us to be the only determinant of the surface properties to be recognized by the macrophage. The fact is that human erythrocytes that have a surface negative charge more than twice as high as that of the rabbit are removed from the circulation within hours. Furthermore, blood cells that are deteriorated during storage in the blood bank show practically no difference in the electric mobility. There is only one paper that reported a slight reduction in the velocity of cells after long storage in a blood bank condition (Ponder and Ponder, 1960). In our experience, there was no modification in electrophoresis of stored erythrocytes. Seaman (personal communication) also found a similar electrophoresis in fresh blood and stored blood. Nevertheless, about 50% of blood stored for 30 days in ACD is removed from the circulation within 24 hours.

CHANGES IN SURFACE ANTIGEN

We have undertaken a very laborious attempt to find out whether there is a specific antigen that is revealed in old cells. Using the differential floatation method after determination of the distribution of specific gravities of the cells (Danon and Marikovsky, 1964), we have separated the one percent oldest cells from rabbit blood and immunized sheep and goats with these cells. After collecting several litres of serum and trying to find a specific antibody to the old cells, we had to admit failure.

Another attempt to reveal a difference in antigenicity was undertaken by electron microscopical methods (Skutelsky et al., 1974). Two immunoferritin techniques (a) ferritin-conjugated antibodies and (b) hybrid antibodies, were used to determine the surface antigen density on separated human young and old erythrocytes and on differentiating rabbit erythroid cells. The alterations of surface antigenicity caused by treatment of erythrocytes with neuraminidase were similarly studied.

It was found that old, untreated cells have about a 25% higher labeling density as compared with the young ones. The same age groups, when treated with neuraminidase, show a 45% increase in labeling density as compared with untreated cells, but without significant differences between young and old cells. Counts performed on cell membranes labeled with ferritin-conjugated antibodies or with hybrid antibodies revealed very similar results with both techniques (figure 6). A progressive increase in labeling density, reaching a maximum at the orthochromatic erythroblast, followed the erythroid cells' division. A slight decrease in antigen density was observed on the reticulocyte. Some cross-reaction with leukoid precursors was also observed. A possible correlation between the reduction of negative surface charge and the increase in membrane antigen density was pointed out.

Expelled erythroid nuclei, surrounded by a narrow rim of cytoplasm and membrane, were found to be more heavily labeled than other erythroid cells of the bone marrow. The increase in antigen density on the membrane surrounding the

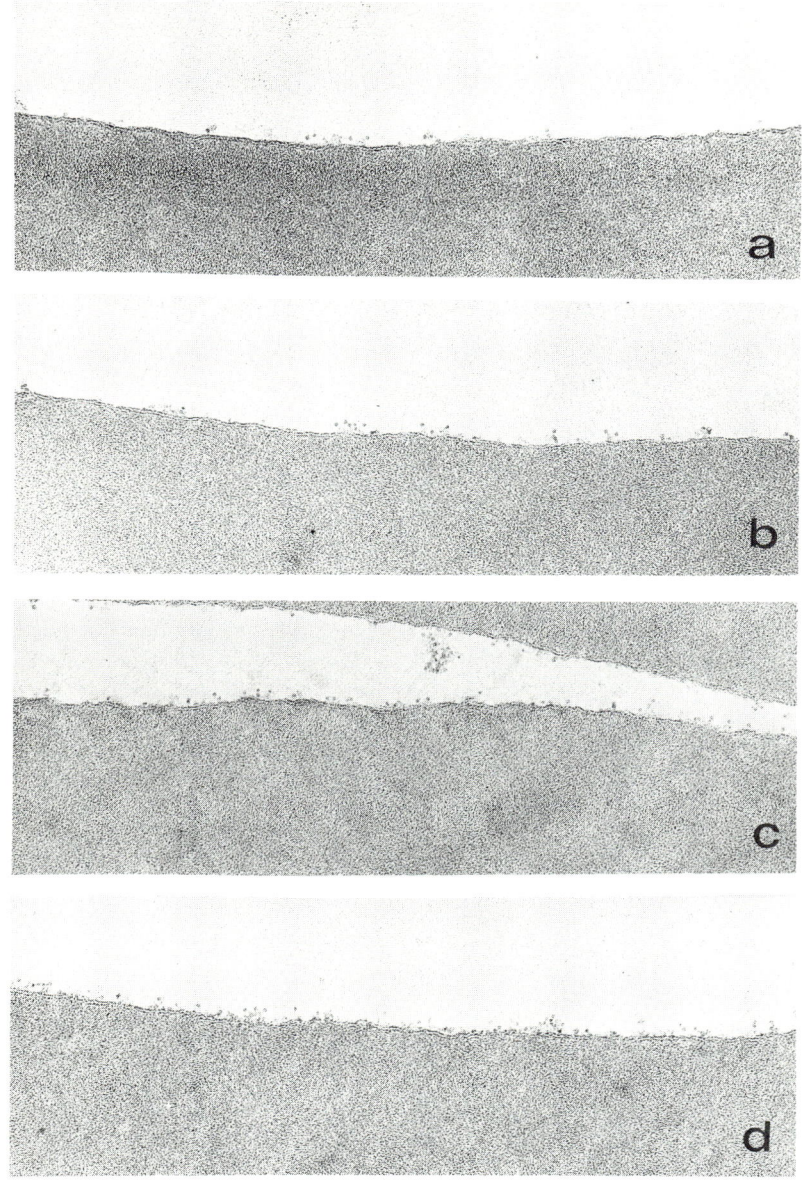

Fig. 6 Human erythrocytes labeled with hybrid antibody ferritin. a) Section of a young erythrocyte. b) Section of an old erythrocyte. c) Section of a young erythrocyte treated with neuraminidase. d) Section of an old erythrocyte treated with neuraminidase. Magnification X100,000. (Skutelsky et al., 1974.)

nucleus is already apparent when the nucleus is partially expelled (figure 7). The alterations in the surface antigen density on old or neuraminidase-treated erythrocytes and on expelled erythroid nuclei are attributed to the appearance of antigens previously masked by the neuraminic acid. It is assumed that the increased membrane antigen density on the surface of old erythrocytes and expelled erythroid nuclei, as well as the reduction in negative surface charge, reflects factors determining the recognition of deteriorated membranes by macrophages and leading to their sequestration.

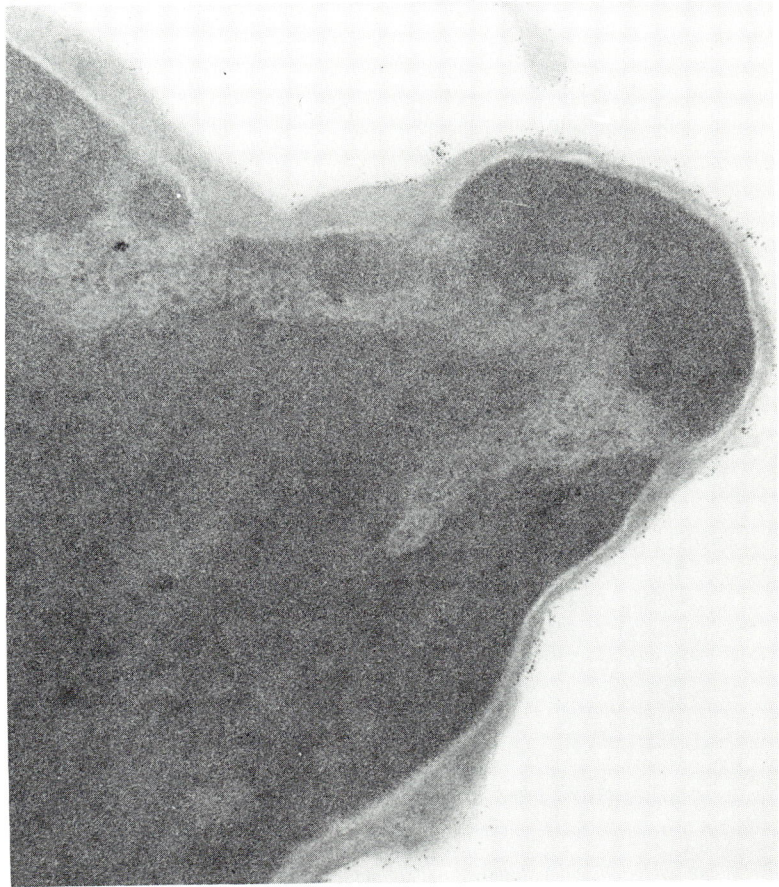

Fig. 7 Orthochromic erythroblast of rabbit bone marrow suspension, treated with goat anti-rabbit erythrocytes-ferritin conjugate. A stage of nuclear expulsion, in which a part of the nucleus is already situated outside the main bulk of the cytoplasm, surrounded ... (continued on page 106)

Fig. 7 (continued) ... by a rim of cytoplasm and cytoplasmic membrane. Note that the part of the membrane surrounding the extruded nucleus (right) is more densely labeled than the parts of the membrane that will remain with the reticulocyte (bottom right and top left). Magnification X50,000. (Skutelsky et al., 1974.)

CONCLUSIONS

It is difficult to ascertain which of the alterations of the surface properties is primarily responsible for the recognition by a macrophage. We think that the diminution in surface charge might be a condition required for closer approach to the cell membranes as well as a recognition sign, but not an exclusive one. The surface antigen newly available for interaction is possibly another sign of recognition which may be considered as a contribution to the understanding of the mechanism by which the macrophage identifies and phagocytizes the deteriorated and undesirable self cells.

REFERENCES

Bessis, M. (1964). In "Ciba Found. Symp. on Cellular Injury" (A.V.S. de Reuck, and J. Knight, eds.), pg. 287, J. A. Churchill Ltd., London.
Brok, F., Ramot, B., Zwang, E., and Danon, D. (1966). Israel J. Med. Sci. 2, 291.
Burton, A. C. (1970). In "Permeability and Function of Biological Membranes" (L. Bolis, A. Katchalsky, R. D. Keynes, W. R. Loewenstein, and B. A. Pethica, eds.), pg. 1, North-Holland Publishing Co., Amsterdam, London.
Danon, D. (1966). Bibliotheca Haematol. 29, 178.
Danon, D., and Marikovsky, Y. (1961). Compt. Rend. CLV, 12.
Danon, D., and Marikovsky, Y. (1964). J. Lab. Clin. Med. 64, 668.
Danon, D., Marikovsky, Y., and Kohn, A. (1969). Experentia 25, 104.
Elazar, E., Marikovsky, Y., and Danon, D. (1971). Unpublished.
Gasko, O., and Danon, D. (1972a). Brit. J. Haematol. 25, 525; 535.
Gasko, O., and Danon, D. (1972b). Exptl. Cell Res. 75, 159.
Gasko, O., and Danon, D. (1974). Brit. J. Haematol. 28, 463.
Gassic, J. G., Berwick, L., and Sorrentino, M. (1968). Lab. Invest. 18, 63.
Gattegno, L., Bladier, D., and Cornillot, P. (1974). Carbohydrate Res. 34, 361.

Halbhuber, K-J., Helmke, U., and Geyer, G. (1972). *Folia Haematol.*, *Leipzig.* 97, 196.
Jancik, J., and Schauer, R. (1974). *Hoppe-Seyler's Z. Physiol. Chem.* 355, 395.
Kent, G., Minik, O. T., Volini, F. I., and Orfei, E. (1966). *Am. J. Pathol.* 48, 831.
Lowenstein, L. M. (1959). *Intern. Rev. Cytol.* 8, 135.
Marikovsky, Y., and Danon, D. (1969). *J. Cell. Biol.* 43, 1.
Marks, P. A. (1961). *Nouvelle Rev. Franc. Hematol.* 1, 900.
Marks, P. A., Rifkind, R. A., and Danon, D. (1963). *Proc. Nat. Acad. Sci. USA*, 50, 336.
Pennel, R. B. (1964). *In* "The Red Blood Cell" (C. Bishop, and D. M. Surgenor, eds.), pg. 20, Academic Press, New York.
Ponder, E., and Ponder, R. V. (1960). *J. Gen. Physiol.* 43, 503.
Schweiger, H. G. (1962). *Intern. Rev. Cytol.* 13, 135.
Skutelsky, E., and Danon, D. (1967). *J. Cell. Biol.* 33, 625.
Skutelsky, E., and Danon, D. (1969). *J. Cell. Biol.* 43, 8.
Skutelsky, E., and Danon, D. (1970). *J. Membrane Biol.* 2, 173.
Skutelsky, E., Marikovsky, Y., and Danon, D. (1974). *Eur. J. Immunol.* 4, 512.
Stephens, J. G. (1940). *J. Physiol.* 99, 30.
Walter, H., Winge, R., and Selby, F. W. (1965). *Biochem. Biophys. Acta* 109, 293.
Weed, R. I., LaCelle, P. L., and Merill, E. V. (1969). *J. Clin. Invest.* 48, 795.
Yaari, A. (1969). *Blood* 33, 159.

CARDIAC CHANGES WITH AGE

Raymond Harris, M.D.

Associate Clinical Professor of Medicine
Albany Medical College
and
Chief, Subdepartment of Cardiovascular Medicine
St. Peter's Hospital
Albany, New York

INTRODUCTION

The biological manifestations of aging as reflected by anatomical, physiological and biochemical alterations in various organs and tissues of the body are responsible for the different clinical manifestations and therapeutic responses between young and old people (Harris, 1970). The sum total of these changes in the heart, attributable to the aging process, constitutes a cardiopathy of aging which can impair cardiac function without clinically evident heart disease. These alterations, whose pathophysiology and biochemistry remain imperfectly understood, appear to develop mainly as a reaction to recurrent hemodynamic stress and the aging process. From evidence obtained by electron microscopy, histochemical, biochemical and other research techniques, this paper discusses the anatomical, physiological and biochemical changes affecting the function of the aging heart in a variety of species.

ANATOMIC CHANGES

Gross changes in the normal aging human heart include alterations in size and geometric contour. The left ventricular cavity tends to become smaller because of the reduced physical demands and activity in old age. Atrophy of the heart may occur in the elderly patient with prolonged illness, confinement to bed, or malnutrition (McKeown, 1965). Enlargement of the left atrium, widening of the aorta as a result of the loss of elasticity, shifting of the aorta to the right, and greater rigidity and thickening of heart valves, place the aged human heart at a mechanical work disadvantage that may impair heart function (Roberts, 1972).

On gross inspection, the aging heart muscle assumes a deeper brown color and the amount of subpericardial fat increases. Fat appears at the entry of the pulmonary veins, the superior vena cava posteriorly, the base of the aorta, and extends from the left circumflex coronary artery upward over the left atrium to involve the region of the sinoatrial node and the intercaval band (Cohn, 1942). Thickened, whitish patches attributable to prolonged hemodynamic stress to which the heart is subjected over the years may be noted in the endocardium, the left atrium, the right atrium, the papillary muscles, and the apical endocardium of the left ventricle. The same, unavoidable hemodynamic stress provokes sclerosis and fibrosis of the valves, causing them to be more rigid and thickened (McMillan and Lev, 1964; Sell and Scully, 1965). The mitral valve is usually more severely affected and its inferior leaflet may show a focal nodularity (Pomerance, 1966). The tricuspid valve and the base of the pulmonic valves may also thicken slightly. Calcification of the aortic valve, starting as a fibrotic thickening on the aortic surface at the base of the cusps, may spread toward the free edges of the cusps as the process progresses.

HISTOLOGIC CHANGES

The atrioventricular valves demonstrate marked disruption of architecture, progressive loss of cellularity, elastosis of the spongiosa and fibrosa, and a marked increase in endocardial hypertrophy. The semilunar valves show similar changes. The aortic valve is more affected than the pulmonic valve, presumably because of the greater hemodynamic stresses to which it is subjected. The aortic leaflets show increased thickness of the noduli and the lines of closure, marked thickening of the base of the aortic cusps, agglutination of the commissures and Lamblian excrescences. Calcium salt deposits associated with arteriosclerosis usually involve the annulus of the valve ring where the adjacent cusps attach, the cusps themselves appearing quite normal (Lev, 1957). Adhesions may be noted at the commissures (Pomerance, 1967). These changes distorting the mitral and aortic valves interfere with their normal closing and create murmurs simulating those produced by more serious acquired heart disease. For example, aging changes in the aortic valve produce a loud aortic systolic murmur which characteristically reaches its maximal intensity during the first half of systole. Fortunately, the hemodynamic consequences of these alterations are usually benign and clinically unimportant, unless organic, acquired valvular disease is also present.

The aging myocardium may also show increased lipochrome pigmentation at the poles of the nuclei of the myocardial fiber, apparent shrinkage and loss of muscle fibers, and focal hypertrophy of the individual fibers. The elastic fibers of the pericardium may increase.

Focal thickening of the elastic and reticular nets and fatty infiltration may be observed in and about the sinoatrial node. Davies and Pomerance (1972) found a significant decrease in the amount of muscle and a corresponding increase in the percentage of fibrous tissue in the sinoatrial node and internodal tracts of patients over 75 years of age at death, as compared with those under 50. They found no increase in adipose tissue within the node. Such changes, starting at about 60 years of age and slowly progressing over the years, may account for the ease with which atrial arrhythmias are induced in old people. Such muscle fiber loss is to be related to either large or small coronary artery disease, since rigid selection of the material excluded coronary atherosclerosis as a factor and the lumen of the sinus node artery itself was larger in old age.

Rakusan and Poupa (1964) compared the number of muscle fibers in hearts of 26- to 27-month old rats with those 4 months of age and found a greater number of muscle fibers per capillary in older animals, which they attributed to greater obliteration of capillaries in the older animals.

Table I summarizes some gross and histologic changes in the aging heart.

ULTRASTRUCTURAL CHANGES

In the Drosophila heart, ultrastructural changes with age include increased size of mitochondria, accumulation of large quantities of intramitochondrial glycogen, increased total extramitochondrial glycogen, development of large autophagic vacuoles, degeneration of nuclei, and the appearance of vacuoles and dense bodies in the sarcoplasm (Burch et al., 1970). The mitochondrial membrane of the myocardium of Drosophila also becomes more abnormal as the fly ages. The mitochondria of the flight muscle of senescent blowflies show accumulation of myelin-like membrane whorls (Smith, 1963) with no cytochrome oxidase activity in nearly 30 percent of the organelles (Sohal, 1970; Sohal and Allison, 1971; Bulos et al., 1972). Similarly, Travis and Travis (1972) reported degenerating forms of mitochondria in the myocardium of old rats.

Table I

Anatomic Changes in the Aging Human Heart*

Changes in size and geometric contour

    Heart size same or smaller
    Smaller left ventricular cavity,
      larger left atrium, dilation of
      aorta as a result of loss of
      elasticity and rightward shift
      of aorta

Endocardial changes

    Thickened whitish patches in
      endocardium, left and right
      atrium, papillary muscles and
      apical endocardium of left
      ventricle

Greater rigidity and thickening of valves

Histologic changes

    Increased collagen in valves
    Increased lipochrome pigmentation
    Increase in elastic fibers of
      pericardium
    Focal thickening of elastic and
      reticular nets and infiltration
      of fat in and about sinoatrial node
    Calcification of media and elastic
      proliferation of musculoelastic
      arteries
    Aging aorta and great vessels -
      increased collagen-elastin ratio
      of aorta and great vessels

---

*Adapted from Harris (1970)

Levkova and Trunov (1970), evaluating by electron microscopy the cardiac mitochondria in 28 albino rats (14 adult and 14 senile), found a decline in the number of mitochondria in the myocardium of old animals. This reduction was attended by an increased volume. They suggest that redox processes decrease in the senile myocardium and that as a result the metabolism of the aged heart may be compelled to convert into an anaerobic route of glycolysis. They believe the myocardium of old animals is probably in a state of high functional stress and vulnerable to sudden physical efforts.

Sanadi (1973) also reports ultrastructural changes in the mitochondrial membrane and a decline in functional integrity with age in more than one species. He confirms that the mitochondrial number per cell may decline in older organisms and postulates such serious limitation in ATP for myocardial activity arising in older animals during periods of high ATP requirement, such as physical exertion and emotional strain, could contribute to cardiac failure.

BIOCHEMICAL CHANGES

Alpert et al. (1967) measured the mechanical and biochemical properties of the hearts of male rats (of the Simonsen strain) ranging in age from 100 to 1000 days and reported a reduction in ATPase activity of fresh myofibrils with age. They noted a significant correlation between the ATPase activity of myofibrils and the velocity of shortening. Their results established an association between contractile protein ATPase activity and velocity of shortening, but not necessarily a cause-and-effect relationship. Furthermore, although the velocity of shortening and the rate of development of isometric force appear to decrease as a function of age, they felt that the ATPase activity of the contractile protein from the heart is age-dependent and that mechanical alterations in function are best related to changes in the ATPase activity rather than to obscure age changes.

These results, showing that velocity of shortening and rate of isometric force development in the myocardium decrease with age, are interpreted to indicate that the heart of old animals must have an active state which develops more slowly, is less intense and is maintained longer than young animals. This type of active state implies age-dependent changes in the ability of the sarcotubular system to remove calcium.

It is well-known that collagen changes qualitatively as a result of greater cross-linking of the collagen macromolecules with age. In addition to these macromolecular changes, the total collagen content of the rat heart may also increase with age. Studying aging of collagen in the heart muscle of 68 female Wistar rats between the ages of one week and 40 months, Schaub (1964-1965) found that the collagen content rises more rapidly than the weight of the ventricular muscles, indicating an active increase of the collagen concentration in the aged rat heart. The total collagen content increased from 1.9 grams per 100 grams of defatted dry tissue in the younger animals to 6.1 in the old.

In the human heart there appears to be no correlation between collagen protein concentration in the left ventricle with age or sex (Blumgart et al., 1940; Wegelius and von Knorring, 1964; Chvapil, 1967) although pathologic processes increased the content of collagen in damaged hearts. Oken and Boucek (1957) noted a higher collagen content in both cardiac ventricles only up to the age of 10. Clausen (1962) found an increase in hydroxyproline content and a decrease in hexosamine concentration during the prenatal and postnatal periods of development. At all ages, the density of collagen connective tissue was higher in the right ventricle than in the left ventricle.

The amount of collagen in the aortic, mitral and tricuspid valves is about 55 percent between the ages of 20 to 30, and decreases by 20 percent in older people. Elastin, constituting about 10 percent of the dried human valve, decreases with age, especially in the mitral and tricuspid valves. The content of acid mucopolysaccharide in the three heart valves also decreases with age, the aortic valve showing the most dramatic reduction (Bashey and Torri, 1965).

The swelling properties of the myocardial proteins of the human heart decrease with age (Kohn and Rollerson, 1959). This decrease may be related to the diminished ability of the aged heart to contract efficiently since swelling ability is a measure of protein elasticity (Limas, 1971). A summary of the changes in myocardial enzymes in the aging heart are shown in Table II.

Sanadi (1973) found the myocardial mitochondria from senescent animals declined in State 3 oxidative rate with certain substrates, but not with others. Chen et al. (1972) interpret these results to "indicate that the control of oxidative metabolism and hence the ATP supply may be altered in aging animals. The magnitude of the decline in State 3 oxidative rates (20-30 percent) may be physiologically significant since this is about the magnitude of change observed in the mitochondria of severely hypothyroid rats. State 3 oxidation represents the maximal rate which would be encountered in vivo only under conditions of extreme energy demand such as strenuous exercise. A decline of 20-30 percent in respiration would decrease ATP production proportionately and impair the energy reserve of older animals for increased cardiac activity and myocardial output to meet stress demands. This in turn could limit oxygen supply to other vital organs with high oxygen demand such as the brain. If, in addition to the decline in mitochondrial oxidative activity, the cells of senescent animals should indeed have fewer mitochondria compared to young adults, the overall decrease in energy production under stress may be seriously inadequate to maintain homeostasis."

Table II

Age-Associated Changes in Myocardial Enzymes*

Enzyme	Type of Change
Monoamine oxidase	Increase
Dopamine β-oxidase	Decrease
Dopa-decarboxylase	Decrease
Catechol-O-methyl transferase	No change
Dopa-α-ketoglutarate transaminase	No change
Lactic dehydrogenase	Decrease
Cytochrome oxidase	Decrease
Succinic oxidase	No change
D-Glucose-6-phosphate dehydrogenase	Decrease
Malic dehydrogenase	Increase
β-Hydroxyacyl-CoA dehydrogenase	No change

*Limas (1971)

PHYSIOLOGIC CHANGES

The effects of aging on the contractile properties of cardiac muscle remain controversial. An increased cardiac pre-ejection period in elderly subjects (Montoye et al., 1971) suggests that the contractility of the myocardium decreases with age. This change possibly may be related to the decreased content of endogenous norepinephrine in the aged myocardium (Gey et al., 1965).

On the other hand, Grodner et al. (1970) conclude that in the rat no deterioration of cardiac muscle contractile function occurs with age. In their study, right ventricular papillary muscles from male Sprague-Dawley rats, aged 150 days, 360 days, 720 days and 1000 days, were suspended in a myograph and stimulated at a frequency of 12/min., producing isometric and variably afterloaded isotonic contractions. Muscle compliance from the length-resting tension relationship was similar for all groups. The velocity of shortening at a preload of 0.6 g/mm^2 was not altered as a function of age. Maximum isometric tension did not diminish with increasing age. Finally, no significant alterations in maximum rate of force development (dp/dt) or time to peak tension (TPT) were noted in the rats up to 720 days old.

Declines in cardiac and stroke volume are not related to differences in sympathetic nervous system tone. Such declines in the rat which has only minimal large vessel coronary atherosclerosis is similar to the decline in these values observed with aging in man (Rothbaum et al., 1973).

Certain physiological changes, as listed in Table III, characterize the aged human heart and impair its function, even in the absence of significant coronary artery disease. For example, the cardiac reserve of the heart and the rate of recovery lessen with age (Harris, 1970). When exercise, emotional stress or other conditions produce tachycardia, the aged myocardium reacts poorly and the senescent patient may show functional cardiac limitations first in normal physiologic stress situations such as exercise or emotional strain and, later, even at rest. Elevated pulse rates of 120 to 150 per minute, produced by simple emotional tachycardia, paroxysmal tachycardia, fever, exercise, or other benign conditions may precipitate heart failure in older people (Dock, 1956). As a result, many older people who can perform normal routine activities, tolerate poorly any of the sudden physical or mental stresses or strains and should be advised against them. Superimposed organic heart diseases may aggravate such changes.

Fortunately, the aged myocardium, despite its decreased power, slow rate of recovery, diminished cardiac reserve and other changes of age usually functions adequately as long as there is sufficient rest between beats. It manages to support an adequate output by prolonging the duration of systole.

Table III

Physiologic Alterations of the
Cardiovascular System With Age*

1. Cardiac output drops 1%/yr below the normal 5 liter/min in younger persons as a result of decreased stroke volume and slower heart rate

2. Estimated left ventricular work declines at rest

3. Maximum blood flow through the coronary artery tree at 60 years of age is about 35% lower than in youth

4. Delay in the recovery of contractility and irritability

5. Cardiac reserve diminishes and heart reacts poorly to sudden stress

6. Normal vasomotor tone decreases; vagal influence increases

7. Peripheral vascular resistance rises 1%/yr

8. Heart less sensitive to atropine and more sensitive to carotid sinus stimulation

9. Decreased ability of heart to utilize oxygen

10. Increased pulse wave velocity

11. Increased cold pressor response

*Adapted from Harris (1970)

The blood pressure in the aging person depends upon the loss of elasticity in the walls of the larger arteries, which tends to raise systolic and depress diastolic pressures and the increased lability of vasopressor control which tends to raise both. These changes increase the rate of rise in pressure (decreased time of arterial upstroke), peak systolic pressure and pulse pressure (Burch and DePasquale, 1969).

With aging, a gradual increase in the irritability of the vasoconstrictor medullary center produced by ischemia, minute arteriosclerotic lesions, or deterioration of specific neuron groups within this area may produce a general vasopressor response which tends to raise the systolic and diastolic blood pressure. Systolic blood pressure usually rises with advancing years; the diastolic pressure may rise or fall (Harris, 1965). Mean systolic blood pressure tends to rise progressively up to the age of 75 to 79. The diastolic pressure tends to rise slightly up to the age of 64 and then gradually declines (Masters and Lasser, 1961).

A practical upper limit of normal blood pressure in the elderly patient is 160 mm Hg systolic and 100 mm Hg diastolic. Increases of 10 to 15 mm Hg in systolic pressure or of 5 mm Hg in diastolic pressure are not alarming and require no drastic treatment or curtailment of the elderly patient's way of life or habits.

The <u>left ventricular ejection</u> time increases 2 milliseconds per decade in the total population, independently of changes in heart rate and blood pressure. A decline in sympathetic nervous tonus and in myocardial contractility and an increase in aortic impedance are probably the main determining factors in prolonging the left ventricular ejection time with age. A decrease of aortic compliance with age is known to increase the impedance to ejection and the tension load on the myocardium independent of changes in aortic pressure (Willems et al., 1970).

CLINICAL EVIDENCE FOR A CARDIOPATHY OF AGING

The preceding data demonstrate definite anatomical, physiological, and biochemical changes in the aging heart of different species. Although no single abnormality is characteristic of the aging process, these cellular, functional, and structural changes provide some insight into the altered functional capacity of the heart in aged animals and humans (Limas, 1971) and support the existence of a cardiopathy of aging.

Can these changes in the aging heart muscle be related to congestive heart failure in old age? As far back as 1945,

Dock postulated that aging of the heart muscle is an important cause of congestive heart failure in old people whose aged myocardium cannot tolerate stresses such as high cardiac output, high arterial pressure, acute febrile illnesses, or tachycardia, without showing signs of heart failure, even in the absence of a specific histologic alteration in the myocardium. He coined the word "presbycardia" to indicate that age alters the ability of the heart to meet its burdens even without significant gross structural abnormalities. Resnik and Harrison (1966) accepted the concept of senile heart disease, classifying it as a primary disorder of cardiac emptying arising from myocardial aging and characterized by the slow onset of heart failure and secondary hypervolemia (Huckabee et al., 1950). Burch and DePasquale (1969) noted elderly patients may develop congestive heart failure and die without any cardiac lesion being found at autopsy sufficient to explain congestive heart failure and death.

However, the clinical evidence for senile heart disease producing congestive heart failure in otherwise normal hearts remains presumptive rather than proven beyond doubt. Heart failure in the aged is usually the result of ordinary pathologic changes such as coronary artery disease, hypertension, valvular disease, or chronic pulmonary lesions. Senile cardiac amyloidosis causes heart failure in a high proportion of elderly patients, as in the case of Pomerance's (1965) study, where it resulted in heart failure in 25 percent of the elderly patients with cardiac decompensation. In all patients with impending or actual myocardial failure, myocarditis and senile heart failure should be considered in the differential diagnosis (Kline et al., 1963). Clinically, myocarditis may be difficult to diagnose in the aged person and is often misdiagnosed as senile cardiopathy. Idiopathic hypertrophic cardiomyopathy, similar to that described in younger people, may occur in the aged (Ohkawa et al., 1971) but should not be confused with senile cardiopathy.

At times, the etiology of heart failure in the elderly remains obscure (Rose and Wilson, 1959). They performed a series of 50 consecutive autopsies on patients over the age of 70 with clinically unexplained heart failure in whom valvular disease, severe coronary artery disease, hypertension, ventricular hypertrophy, anemia, pulmonary emphysema, malnutrition, thyrotoxicosis, or cardiac failure as a terminal complication of pneumonia or of surgical procedures were excluded. Three possible causes of heart failure in these patients were postulated by these workers, as follows:

1. hypertension which had decreased due to failure,

2. myocardial ischemia, and

3. a degenerative process associated with aging.

Although ischemia is widely held to cause most cases of clinically obscure cardiac failure, Rose and Wilson (1959), finding ischemic changes in 38 percent of controls, concluded that diffuse fibrosis was almost equally frequent in patients with or without heart failure. Pomerance (1965) found "senile heart failure" or congestive failure uncommon for patients with completely normal hearts, in her series involving 370 subjects over the age of 75. There were only 7 cases (2 percent) in the category of "senile heart failure", and anemia probably accounted for heart failure in three of these cases. Although brown atrophy is sometimes thought to be responsible for failure in the elderly, Dr. Pomerance's experience with large numbers of elderly hearts confirmed the findings of Rose and Wilson (1959) that brown atrophy is more common in hearts of patients without cardiac failure and is generally seen only in small hearts such as those of patients dying of carcinomatosis or other wasting disease. It is noteworthy that the small heart is less likely to go into congestive failure despite its brown atrophy (Sonnek, 1954).

Although there is evidence for a cardiopathy of aging due to the anatomical, biochemical and physiological changes demonstrated in the aging myocardium, there is still insufficient evidence to link the so-called senile cardiopathy of aging directly to otherwise unexplained heart failure in the aged. More needs to be learned about the subcellular, molecular morphology and molecular biology of the aging process in the human heart of patients with and without heart failure.

In our present state of knowledge, otherwise unexplained heart failure in aged people may be attributed to a clinicophysiologic senile heart failure syndrome which is associated with depression of intrinsic myocardial function. In the failing heart, the rate of converting energy to work at a normal efficiency is decreased, probably as a result of reduced activity of myofibrillar adenosine triphosphatase, which may be causally related to depressed cardiac function (Pool and Braunwald, 1968). Geometric changes in ventricular size, shape, wall thickness, or asynchrony of contraction reduces the efficiency of the senile heart. Finally, since the failing heart depends on supporting mechanisms, such as adrenergic stimulation for normal function, the reduced intrinsic norepinephrine stores in the aged myocardium and the amount of circulating catecholamines may be important factors in the development of senile heart failure. Eventually, a specific involutional change may be identified in the myocardium of the aged person with heart failure. If so, an additional pathologic condition -- senile heart disease -- may be added to the already accepted etiologic causes of acquired heart disease in old age.

REFERENCES

Alpert, N., Gale, H., and Taylor, N. (1967). In "Factors Influencing Myocardial Contractility" (R. D. Tanz, ed.), pp. 127-133, Academic Press, New York.
Bashey, R. I., and Torri, S. (1965). Abstract, 18th Annual Meeting, Gerontological Society, Los Angeles, California.
Blumgart, H. L., Gilligan, D. R., and Schlesinger, M. J. (1940). Trans. Assoc. Am. Physicians 55, 313.
Bulos, B., Shukla, S., and Sacktor, B. (1972). Arch. Biochem. Biophys. 149, 461.
Burch, G., and DePasquale, N. (1969). Am. Heart J. 78, 700.
Burch, G., Sohal, R. S., and Fairbanks, L. D. (1970). Nature 225, 286.
Chen, J. C., Warshaw, J. B., and Sanadi, D. R. (1972). J. Cell. Physiol. 80, 141.
Chvapil, M. (1967). "Physiology of Connective Tissue". Czechoslovak Medical Press, Butterworth and Co., London.
Clausen, B. (1962). Lab. Invest. 11, 229.
Cohn, A. E. (1942). In "Problems of Ageing" (E. V. Cowdry, ed.), pp. 111-138, Williams and Wilkins, Baltimore.
Davies, M. J., and Pomerance, A. (1972). Brit. Heart J. 34, 150.
Dock, W. (1945). N.Y. State J. Med. 45, 983.
Dock, W. (1956). Bull. N.Y. Acad. Med. 32, 175.
Gey, K. F., Burkard, W. P., and Pletscher, A. (1965). Gerontologia 11, 1.
Grodner, A., Pool, P., and Braunwald, E. (1970). Abstracts of 43rd Scientific Sessions, American Heart Association. Supp. to Circulation, Vol. XLI and XLII, October, p.115.
Harris, R. (1965). In "Clinical Features of the Older Patient" (J. T. Freeman, ed.), pp. 125-137, Charles C Thomas, Springfield, Illinois.
Harris, R. (1970). "The Management of Geriatric Cardiovascular Disease". J. B. Lippincott Co., Philadelphia.
Huckabee, W., Casten, G., and Harrison, T. (1950). Circulation 1, 343.
Kline, I., Kline T., and Saphir, O. (1963). Am. Heart J. 65, 446.
Kohn, R., and Rollerson, E. (1959). Proc. Soc. Exptl. Biol. 100, 253.

Lev, M. (1957). Military Med. 120, 257.
Levkova, N. A., and Trunov, V. I. (1970). Kardiologiia 10, 94.
Limas, C. J. (1971). Acta Cardiol. 26, 249.
Masters, A. M., and Lasser, R. P. (1961). In "Hypertension: Recent Advances" (A. M. Brest and J. H. Moyer, eds.), pp. 24-34, Lea and Febiger, Philadelphia.
McKeown, F. (1965). "Pathology of the Aged". Butterworth, London.
McMillan, J., and Lev, M. (1964). J. Gerontol. 19, 1.
Montoye, H. J., Willis, P. W.,III, Howard, G. E., and Keller, J. B. (1971). J. Gerontol. 26, 208.
Ohkawa, S., Sugiura, M., Ilizuka, T., Shimada, H., and Okada, R. (1971). Japan. Heart J. 12, 305.
Oken, D. E., and Boucek, R. J. (1957). Circulation Res. 5, 357.
Pomerance, A. (1965). Brit. Heart J. 27, 697.
Pomerance, A. (1966). Brit. Heart J. 28, 815.
Pomerance, A. (1967). Brit. Heart J. 29, 222.
Pool, P., and Braunwald, E. (1968). Am. J. Cardiol. 22, 7.
Rakusan, K., and Poupa, O. (1964). Gerontologia 9, 107.
Resnik, W. H., and Harrison, T. R. (1966). In "Principles of Internal Medicine" (T. R. Harrison, R. D. Adams, I. L. Bennett, W. H. Resnik, G. W. Thorn, and M. M. Wintrobe, eds.), 5th edition, pp. 733-735, The Blakiston Division, McGraw-Hill Book Co., New York.
Roberts, W. C. (1972). Personal communication.
Rose, G. A., and Wilson, R. R. (1959). Brit. Heart J. 21, 511.
Rothbaum, D. A., Shaw, D. J., Angell, C. S., and Shock, N. W. (1973). J. Gerontol. 28, 287.
Sanadi, D. R. (1973). In "Myocardial Metabolism" (N. S. Dhalla, ed.), Vol. 3, pp. 91-96, University Park Press, Baltimore.
Schaub, M. C. (1964-1965). Gerontologia 10, 38.
Sell, S., and Scully, R. E. (1965). Am. J. Pathol. 46, 345.
Smith, D. S. (1963). J. Cell Biol. 19, 115.
Sohal, R. S. (1970). Exp. Gerontol. 5, 213.
Sohal, R. S., and Allison, V. F. (1971). Exp. Gerontol. 6, 167.
Sonnek, P. J. (1954). Geriatrics 9, 75.
Travis, D. F., and Travis, A. (1972). J. Ultrastruct. Res. 39, 124.
Wegelius, O., and von Knorring, J. (1964). Acta Med. Scand. 175, Suppl. 233.
Willems, J. L., Roelandt, J., DeGeest, H., Kesteloot, H., and Joossens, J. V. (1970). Circulation XLII, 37.

ATHERO-ARTERIOSCLEROSIS AS AN AGING PHENOMENON

Herman T. Blumenthal

Aging and Development Program
Department of Psychology
Washington University
St. Louis, Missouri 63130

Delineation of the Problem

It is evident from vital statistics of the past 25 years that degenerative vascular disease is the most prevalent disorder after about age 45, and remains so after age 65 (U. S. Dept. HEW Publ. # (HSM) 72-1207). However, the magnitude of the problem is not as clear. There are differences between crude and age-adjusted rates, but perhaps an even greater confounding factor is the manner in which causes of death are listed. One finds among the leading causes of death "diseases of the heart" (presumably including ischemic heart disease, myocardial infarction, etc.) and "cerebrovascular disease" (presumably cerebral hemorrhage or infarction), as well as "diabetes mellitus", "hypertension" and "arteriosclerosis". The latter three designations obscure more than they reveal. The vast majority of deaths associated with maturity-onset diabetes are due to myocardial infarction, stroke, gangrene of the lower extremity or diabetic nephropathy, rather than to chemical effects linked with diabetes. A similar argument can be made in respect to hypertension in which death is most often linked with myocardial infarction, stroke or uremia from vascular renal disease. The separate listing of arteriosclerosis does not delineate whether death is due to myocardial infarction, stroke, gangrene of the extremity, vascular renal disease, aneurysm of the aorta, etc.

The problem is further confounded by the assumption of certain cause and effect relationships. One such assumption is that coronary artery thrombosis or occlusion causes myocardial infarction, and one often reads that there is a "modern epidemic" of deaths due to ischemic heart disease. An objective assessment of the available data indicates that in all probability more patients have myocardial infarction without acute coronary artery thrombosis than with a thrombus, and indeed it has even been suggested that infarction may precede and cause the thrombosis (Robbins, 1974; Warren, 1973). Anderson (1970) suggests that the rise in the male death rate from ischemic heart disease over the past 50 years has been due to an increased tendency of the myocardium to infarction rather than to an increased tendency to intravascular thrombosis.

Several years ago I expressed concern regarding the deliberations of a National Heart and Lung Institute (NHLI) Task Force on Arteriosclerosis because gerontology was not represented (Blumenthal, 1972). In its subsequent report (U. S. Dept. HEW Publ. # (NIH) 72-137) in which it largely proposed another decade or two of research along the same lines as in the two preceding decades, this task force essentially ignored aging as a significant factor in the genesis of arteriosclerosis. It is especially not clear from the NHLI Report whether the recommendations are intended to deal with the genesis of arteriosclerosis or with certain related problems such as myocardial infarction, stroke, etc. To avoid this ambiguity it is the intention here to restrict this presentation to a consideration of concepts dealing with the genesis of athero-arteriosclerosis (AA). The reason for selecting the latter terminology is noted below.

Some Historical Perspective

Page (1974) has recently noted that "far too many physicians and scientists, as well as laymen, look upon the history of discovery as an entertaining pastime, a tiresome academic exercise, or merely the record of egotistical aspirations ..... Today many investigators fail to appreciate that knowledge of the history of discovery is vital if wise policies are to be generated". It might be suggested that if the NHLI Task Force had seriously taken into account the total history of information regarding arteriosclerosis rather than just the antecedent several decades, it might have reached different conclusions. For example, the much heralded epidemic of ischemic heart disease may not be what it seems. Arteriosclerosis has proved to be a common finding in Egyptian mummies, and there is evidence that this vascular disorder was at least as common among the Egyptians and their neighbors as it is today, and possibly even exceeded the modern incidence (Long, 1967).

Table I provides a list of risk factors for ischemic heart disease from the Task Force Report. It is an interesting exercise to apply these to ancient Egyptian society. For example, the Egyptians evidently did not smoke cigarettes,

and considering modes of transportation, the organization of
their society and the characteristics of their industries,
most probably did not lack exercise; moreover, their
emotional stresses were probably quite different from ours.
There is also a considerable likelihood that the fat content
of their diet was significantly different from ours since
they depended largely on grain and fruit, with meat probably
reserved for ritual occasions. While the Bible relates the
tending of small flocks, it provides no evidence that they
engaged in the currently common practice of fattening animals
for market to enhance their commercial value.

Table I

Major Risk Factors in Athero-Arteriosclerosis*

Dietary intake of lipids and serum cholesterol
Hypertension
Cigarette smoking
Diabetes and impaired glucose tolerance
Familial and genetic factors
Obesity
Lack of exercise
Male predominance
Emotional stress
Softness of drinking water
Elevated blood uric acid

(AGING ?)#

---

*From National Heart and Lung Institute Task
  Force on Arteriosclerosis
#Our addition

Arteriosclerosis Research. According to the eminent
pathologist-historian Long (1967), our knowledge of the
existence of arteriosclerosis dates from the relatively
crude observations of the anatomists of the 16th century;
this was soon accepted as a natural phenomenon related to
the "advance of life" - i.e., an aging phenomenon. As Long
(1967) further indicated, most early observers emphasized
the rigid, hard quality of the artery wall until von Haller
(1751) directed attention to soft mushy areas. Although the
term atheroma designating these soft spots was first introduced by Marchand (1904), it was Klotz (1911) who argued
that it should be restricted to intimal changes.
    The idea that intimal plaques result from excessive
deposits of material from the blood mass was first introduced

by Rokitansky (1841) and persists today in explaining the entry of lipids into the intima to initiate the formation of atheromatous plaques. On the other hand, it was Virchow (1856) who proposed that after an initial loosening of ground substance intimal cells undergo an almost neoplastic proliferation before degenerative changes set in, and he emphasized further that these changes occur in regions where the force of the blood stream is such as to lend to pressure and thickening. However, delineation of the role of mechanical factors in the distribution of lesions should be credited to Thoma (1861); he proposed that intimal proliferation represents a compensatory process to vascular dilatation, and since medial degeneration is a progressive continuing process, the demand for intimal proliferation should thereby also be progressive and continuing.

According to Long (1967), historically three basic concepts developed with respect to the etiology of this phenomenon; aging, an inflammatory genesis, and abnormalities in lipid metabolism. Aging was considered to be a primary factor until well into the 20th century. As already noted, Thoma placed the role of aging in the context of mechanical wear and tear, and this concept was taken up by Klotz (1911), Ophuls (1921) and Aschoff (1933). The possibility of an inflammatory genesis was raised by Hodgson (1815) and taken up later by Winternitz and associates (1938), Karsner (1937) and in more recent years by Saphir (1964). A lipid genesis first received serious consideration around 1910 following a series of studies by Ignatowsky and by Saltykow in which diets rich in cow's milk and egg yolk resulted in the formation of lipid deposits in the aorta of rabbits. But it was Anitschkow who ultimately laid down the dictum that increased cholesterol in the blood is the exciting cause of atherosclerosis, the others serving only as predisposing factors. With some modification, this remains the dominant current view. Motivated by the poor correlation in humans between cholesterolemia and vascular disease, Gofman and associates (1950) emphasized the role of circulating giant lipoprotein molecules as the carriers of the lipids deposited in arteries.

The above historical summary drawn primarily from Long's (1967) account serves to emphasize the complexity of the lesion. Intimal mounds in rather specific locations have been considered to be either deposits from the blood mass, or multiple benign tumors. Degenerations of vascular tissues with focal areas of calcification within the wall have been considered separate wear and tear effects, and inflammatory cell infiltrates have been attributed to irritant effects of lipid deposits. Arteriosclerosis has come to be applied as the term covering all non-lipid phenomena and considered largely to be an aging phenomenon of little clinical importance. Atherosclerosis has emerged as the term representing the intimal changes considered to be primarily responsible for narrowing of the lumen of arteries and subsequent thrombosis. Nevertheless, ambiguity of terminology remains. Thus, the NHLI Task Force, cited above, entitles its report as dealing with arteriosclerosis, but the text often refers to atheroma formation and atherosclerosis. To emphasize the fact that there may be a unifying concept which includes all components of the artery lesion, we have combined the two in the terminology "athero-arteriosclerosis", rather awkward in form but which, at least, can be abbreviated conveniently as AA.

The Pathology of Normalcy

The heading of this section has been borrowed from a chapter in Erich Fromm's "The Sane Society" (1955), entitled "Can A Society be Sick? - The Pathology of Normalcy". The analagous question here is "Does a society of aged people succumb to a normal process or a disease?" Most investigators, whether in gerontology or some other medical science, have been operating on a schizophrenoid principle which separates so-called "normal aging" from disease. For example, Andres (1973) has noted that if we apply the same diagnostic criteria for diabetes mellitus to a population over age 65 as we do to a population under age 30, then a very large percent of the old people would have diabetes. Since most investigators find such a conclusion unacceptable, they consider the manifestations of diabetes in many of the aged to represent normal senescence.

Aging, while generally conceded to be deleterious to the organism, is separated from disease on the basis that it is an intrinsic universal phenomenon which is genetically programmed. Disease, on the other hand, is considered to have a primary environmental cause, with aging playing only a secondary role, either in the form of increasing vulnerability, or by virtue of permitting a sufficiently long exposure to environmental agents requiring long latent periods. Universality implies that in the absence of disease, individuals of all species who live long enough should ultimately succumb to the same biological phenomenon. It essentially ignores the fact that evolution has introduced a considerable number of adaptive phenomena which may modify such a basic process in a variety of ways including its time of appearance and its manifestations. It may be significant that the same Gompertz equation which expresses mortality in the absence of disease in animals low on the phylogenetic tree also applies to death as a consequence of disease in mammals. The relation of genetic programming to disease is discussed in a later section.

The issue of prevalence as implied by universality can be a misleading one. On the one hand, as Dubois (1968) has noted, there have been some societies in the past in which tuberculosis was so common as to be considered "normal". This concept, of course, disappeared with the discovery of the causal organism. On the other hand, for almost a quarter of a century we have been pursuing a lipid-metabolic causation of AA. There have been a multitude of studies attempting to relate blood levels of various lipid components to incidence, utilizing even more sophisticated analytic techniques. Others have attempted to correlate incidence with the dietary characteristics of various ethnic and racial populations. There have been animal experiments with numerous types of dietary manipulations, and human studies directed at manipulating diets to prevent or retard progress of the disorder. Most recently, there has even been some emphasis on initiating dietary prevention in infancy based largely on the presence of lipid streaks in the aortas of children. In addition, there are programs aimed at removing or controlling the various risk factors in Table I.

The inconclusive character of these programs can be appreciated from the fact that, in one form or another, they have been promoted for over two decades without significant impact on mortality rates, and from the fact that the NHLI Task Force has recommended that they be continued for at least another decade or two, while at the same time making no new recommendations for studies on primary etiology. The Coronary Drug Project, a nationwide study begun in 1966 and sponsored by NHLI at a cost of $40 million, is another example of an inconclusive study (Blumenthal, 1972). Several drugs known to have a serum cholesterol lowering effect have been shown to have no influence on decreasing the risk of having a heart attack or of prolonging the lives of those who have already had one. Nevertheless, two accomplishments have been emphasized: 1) the project shows the feasibility of large scale cooperative ventures, and 2) the clinicians discovered a great deal about predicting a patient's progress after a heart attack. This inability to admit failure and to turn attention to the pursuit of alternative concepts might be considered by some to be symptomatic of "Future Shock". The hazard inherent in this rigidity is that after another two decades of current lines of research on AA, we may be no closer to an understanding of the problem than at present.

In practice, opinions regarding the aging-disease relationship appears to be based more on an understanding of etiology than on the issues of universality and genetic programming. This is implied in the expression "Infinitely Eliminable" as applied by Kleemeier (1965). His basic point is that as the etiology of a disorder previously considered to be due to aging is identified so that it becomes possible to conceptualize definitive preventive or therapeutic modes, the phenomenon is transferred from the status of an aging process to one of disease. If this process is carried to its extreme, all disorders at one time considered to be due to aging would eventually become preventable or curable diseases, and there would no longer be a need for gerontology as a discipline. AA appears to have progressed through this process. Once considered to be an aging phenomenon, it is currently viewed by most investigators and clinicians as a lipid-metabolic disease, and preventive and therapeutic measures are primarily directed at this etiology. But the announcement of the death of aging in the causation of AA may be premature. Despite a mass of statistical studies, age remains the best correlate with the incidence and severity of this vascular disorder.

Error - Autoimmune Theory of Aging and Disease

It has recently been noted that there are about as many theories of aging as there are biologists engaged in research in aging (Marx, 1975). For the past decade, we have been examining the possibility that two currently popular theories of aging may be combined into a single concept which would account for the prevalence of certain diseases of the aged as a direct extension of certain fundamental biological aging phenomena. If this concept can be proved valid, then the aging-disease relationship would be a causal rather than a casual one.

As Wilson (1974) has pointed out, there are "how" and "why" theories of aging. The "how" theories can be placed in three groups:

1. The playing out of genetic program - an extension of embryological moulding.

2. The expression of specific genes for aging.

3. The accumulation of errors or misinformation in information-containing molecules.

Gerontologists have long recognized that as cells age they accumulate a variety of substances not present in young cells. When such substances are proteins to which the immune system did not have access during embryogenesis, they are dealt with by the adult organsim as "not-self". Thus, the products of genes derepressed late in life, whether as a consequence of the running out of genetic program or the expression of specific genes from aging, would have this characteristic. The several so-called fetal antigens which appear in adult cells fall into this category. There are several variations of error theory, including a currently popular one termed "error catastrophe" as proposed by Orgel (1973). Generally not considered by error theorists is the additional possibility that mis-specification deriving from mitochondrial DNA may contribute to error accumulation as well as that deriving from nuclear DNA. One consequence of such phenomena has recently been summarized by Goldstein (1974) as follows: "Recent work indicates that cells undergoing aging accumulate a multiplicity of abnormal gene products that almost certainly represent molecular mischief one or more steps removed from the primary events. In any case the spatiotemporal relationships within and between cells, organized as multitiered feedback loops orchestrating cellular function into an efficient bodily whole, begin to break down. In the language of communications, the 'signal-to-noise' ratio decreases. Compensatory increases in signal output ultimately lead to intensified noise production and finally systems failure".

This brief description of error effects by Goldstein may account for many of the physiological deficits characteristic of aging, as well as for some of the compensatory processes. However, it omits one essential consideration. Higher organisms possess an immune system capable of removing cells possessing not-self antigens and thereby also eliminating interfering "noise". Many current investigations deal with this concept in respect to the control of the deviant cancer cell, but it may also have applicability to aging cells more generally. Ultimately, however, cells of the immune system seem to fall prey to the same error phenomena as cells of other organ systems.

To account for the consequences of such immune system failure, Burnet (1973) has proposed a "why" theory which places aging in an evolutionary context. He notes that the program for each mammalian species provides for the greatest survival potential during the years of maximum reproductive capacity, for the human roughly between 15 and 30 years of age. Burnet notes further that the mortality curve is bimodal, with a minor peak between birth and 15 years and an ascending curve representing a progressively increasing mortality rate beginning at age 30. The programming of the immunosurveillance system appears to determine this survival potential. From birth to age 15 it is in process of development, but not yet at optimum efficiency; hence the minor mortality peak. After age 30, it progressively loses efficiency as documented by Adler (1974). While most physicians recognize that this bimodal curve is applicable to neoplasms, diabetes, rheumatoid arthritis and several other disorders in which there are juvenile and adult or maturity-onset forms, it is not generally appreciated that it also applies to cardiovascular disease as illustrated in figure 1. The juvenile forms can probably be attributed to inherited genetic defects, while the maturity-onset forms may derive from an aging-acquired gene disorder in accordance with the various "how" theories. What is particularly noteworthy is that at least the second segment of this curve also applies to the incidence of so-called non-disease deteriorations of non-mammalian as well as mammalian species, including humans.

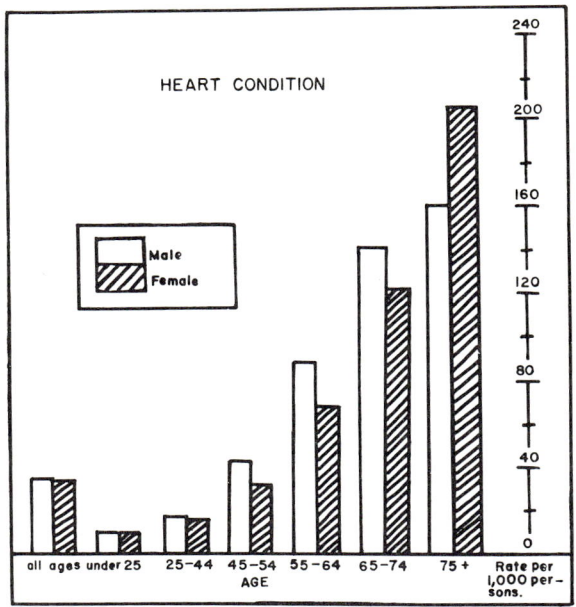

Fig. 1 Incidence of cardiovascular disease. From health statistics from the U. S. National Health Surveys, Series B-No. 13 (Hilleboe, 1967).

As Shock (1974) has noted, at least some of the foregoing hypotheses are currently testable. At the cellular level much of this testing involves the use of an experimental model deriving from the discovery of Hayflick and Morehead (1961) that cultured embryo fibroblasts have a finite number of doubling generations which roughly corresponds to the life span of the species from which they are derived. The evidence in respect to the accumulation of errors in late doubling generations is presently inconclusive, but heteroploid cells of varying growth potential seem to occur in these cultures and some of the latter give rise to permanent immortal lines analagous to cancer. There are some observations which are relevant to the genesis of AA as discussed below. These are as follows:

1. Not all cells capable of mitotic division are committed simultaneously. The organism possesses resting pools of stem cells with reservoir function which become committed either on a programmed basis or on special demand.

2. The life span of diploid cells is probably more closely related to the number of cell or population doublings than to chronological time. In fibroblast cultures, the doubling time increases and mitotic activity decreases in late doubling generations. Moreover, cultures can be manipulated to increase the number of cells in a lag or stationary phase which later can be reactivated.

3. Gelfant and Grove (1974) have reported that the proportion of non-dividing cells increase to about 48 percent in late doubling generations when the percent of incorporation of H^3-thymidine decreases. They interpret these findings as indicating that in early passages a large proportion are synthesizing DNA. Thus, in early passages, most non-dividing cells are G_1 blocked, while in late passages they are G_2 blocked, and many of the latter are polyploid. Moreover, the potential for release from non-cycling to cycling diminishes with the age of the culture.

4. Holliday (1975) has raised some important questions in relation to these heteroploid cells. Can diploids give rise to heteroploid cells with equal frequency at all phases of growth? Gelfant and Grove's observations (1974) indicate that they occur more frequently in late phases. What proportion of the

heteroploid cells produce a permanent immortal line, and how many still show senescence? While our own studies, noted in sections which follow, do not shed light on the frequency with which heteroploid cells give rise to hyperplasias, benign tumors or cancers, they do indicate that in some organ systems, at least, heteroploidy, hyperplasia and benign tumors are frequent concomitants of aging.

5. Late passage cells contain enzymes with higher temperature lability and lower specific activity than early passage cells, and exhibit changes in their interactions with polymerizing fibrin. In a more general vein, there are alterations in late passage cultures which may relate to self-recognition and certain autoimmune concomitants of aging *in vivo* including atherothrombosis and diabetes. Not only is the number of doubling generations of cultured fibroblasts reduced in such disorders as progeria, Werner's syndrome and diabetes mellitus, but a number of these abnormal late phase concomitants also occur in earlier doubling generations (Goldstein et al., 1975; Vracko and Benditt, 1975).

As Shock (1974) has already remarked, there is a considerable gap between cell culture studies and aging in a total animal. In particular, it should be noted that the time at which heteroploid or senescent cells might be present in sufficient number to give rise to disease is highly dependent upon modulating, inhibiting, stimulating and censoring influence of the neuroendocrine and immune systems. For about a decade (and preceding the current interest in the Hayflick phenomenon), we have been engaged in an attempt to correlate several aging phenomena demonstrable by histo- and immunopathological techniques with diseases of aging in the context of error-autoimmune theory. These phenomena are as follows:

1. The appearance of dyskaryotic nuclei.

2. The occurrence of adenomatous hyperplasia.

3. The infiltration of lymphoid cells into areas with dyskaryotic nuclei and adenomatous hyperplasia.

4. The deposition of hyaline and/or amyloid in the absence of lymphoid cell infiltration.

5. The dissemination of a proliferative vascular lesion associated with autoimmune states.

For the most part, our investigations in this regard have centered about the endocrine system, and largely in respect to an autoimmune genesis of diabetes (Blumenthal, 1971). The appearance of dyskaryotic cells and foci of adenomatous hyperplasia have been considered to represent clones of deviant (mis-specified) cells, and the lymphocytic infiltration as an expression of immunosurveillance. The ultimate replacement of parenchymal elements by hyaline or amyloid deposits have been regarded as evidence of failure of the immunosurveillance mechanism.

In addition to the changes in the endocrine glands, we have also described a disseminated angiopathy characterized by a proliferation of intimal cells which we regarded as endothelial (Blumenthal, 1968). Several of these studies dealt with this vascular lesion in relation to maturity-onset diabetes in which the islets of Langerhans often exhibit certain of the histopathological lesions noted above, but there were also observations reported which suggest that this angiopathy is associated with other phenomena of possible autoimmune origin.

While current cell culture studies provide an opportunity for testing error theory at the cellular level, they also provide an opportunity for evaluating certain aging phenomena and diseases of aging in the total organism when correlated with certain aging changes in organ systems. In the remainder of this presentation, we shall deal with the Hayflick phenomenon as it may relate to the genesis of AA.

The Origin of Intimal Plaques

It is perhaps ironic that after about 75 years of dominance of the concept that atheroma derive from a reaction of intimal tissues to the deposition of lipids, there is again serious consideration of Virchow's proposal of 1856 that intimal plaques may represent foci of neoplastic proliferation. In a sense, our studies (Blumenthal, 1968) dealing with an autoimmune proliferative angiopathy might be construed as supporting Virchow's view, although these observations were not generalized to include the larger problem of AA. In any event, even such a limited concept of the participation of vascular elements in immune responses was not generally accepted. Recently, however, Benditt and Benditt (1973) have again proposed that intimal plaques may be benign tumors, but deriving from repeated reproduction of a single abnormal intimal smooth muscle cell. While these investigators appear to favor a chemical mutagen, virus or physical agent in the causation of such a phenomenon, their studies by no means eliminate the possibility of an aging process in the context of the Hayflick model. In fact, Martin and Sprague (1974), working in the same department as the Benditts, have proposed that atherogenesis may be related to the limited replication life span of intimal smooth muscle cells, and Vracko and Benditt (1974) have proposed the acceleration of such a process in diabetes.

Martin and Sprague (1974) propose that in vivo there is normally a negative feedback inhibition which controls the growth of intimal smooth muscle cells and that dormant stem cells undergo activation and clonal senescence when released from this inhibition. They propose further that at sites more prone to plaque formation there may be an increased tendency to undergo such a release. However, there are several other mechanisms which merit consideration. One possibility is that the heteroploid cells which develop during clonal senescence exhibit not-self characteristics and evoke an immune response similar to that observed in vessels following homografting. However, there are paradoxical aspects in respect to immune responses which are comparable to those observed with tumors more generally. On the one hand, T lymphocytes may home in and attack such deviant cells, while on the other, circulating antibodies may coat cell surfaces, protecting them from T cell attack, and permitting their continuing growth. There is evidence that both these immune processes take place in blood vessels. Figure 2 shows a proliferation of intimal cells, with some cells showing nuclear enlargement suggestive of heteroploidy. The adjacent lymphocytic infiltration is indicative of the homing in of T cells. Figure 3 is illustrative of the coating of intimal cells by immunoglobulins.

One critical aspect of dealing with differences in the behavior of intimal cells as between sites of low and high predilection for plaque formation is whether the observed differences represent cause or effect. It would appear that differences in biochemical characteristics as well as in immune reactions are more likely to represent effects relating to clonal senescence, while the activation of stem cells and the acceleration of clonal senescence can be more directly related to hemodynamic factors as detailed in the section immediately following.

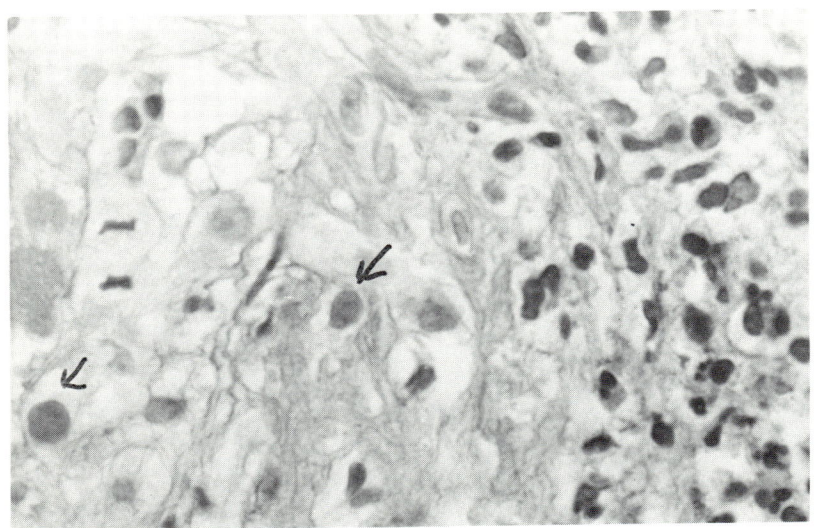

Fig. 2 Intima of anterior tibial artery of 72-year-old male. H and E stain; mag. approx. 500X. Mitotic figure is near left margin and infiltrating lymphocytes along right margin. Arrows indicate dyskaryotic cells.

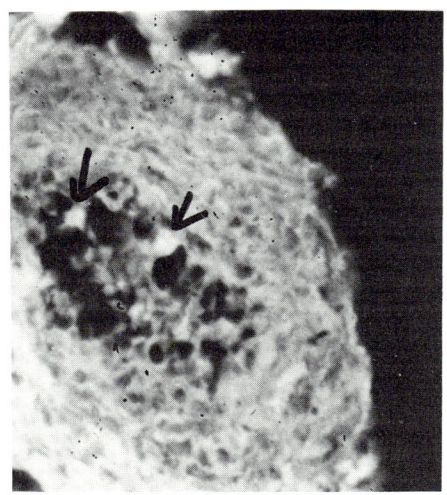

Fig. 3 Cross section of anterior tibial artery from same case as figure 2. "Stained" with fluorescein-tagged rabbit anti-human gamma globulin and photographed with ultra-violet light. Mag. approx. 100X. Arrows indicate brightly fluorescent intimal cells.

The Role of Hemodynamic Factors in the Localization and Genesis of Intimal Plaques

We have reviewed elsewhere (Blumenthal, 1967) a considerable body of data deriving from the studies of Burton (1951) and of Texon (1963) which show that the anatomic distribution of plaques can best be accounted for on the basis of hemodynamic forces which are intensified at sites of predilection because of special physical features which obtain at these locations, particularly as they relate to local blood pressure and lumen radius. There are also data which support the concept that there is a basic structural homeostasis which the organism strives to maintain during its life span. The latter can be expressed as a wall thickness-internal diameter (WT/ID) ratio. As an artery dilates with age, probably as a consequence of wear and tear effects of hemodynamic forces on vascular tissue components, the intimal elements proliferate until the ratio is reestablished. Ultimately, as with other homeostatic mechanisms, this one also loses efficiency with advancing age and failure can be recognized either in the form of a disproportionate narrowing of the lumen and even its complete closure, or conversely in aneurysm formation.

The proliferative process can be uniform and symmetrical along the internal circumference of an artery when hemodynamic forces are applied equally in all directions, or there may be asymmetric foci when such forces are applied unequally because of particular anatomic characteristics such as focal widening at the origin of branches, the development of tortuosities, or other sites of particular stress.

It would appear that this concept can now be applied to the activation of stem cells to undergo clonal senescence, with the latter process serving to maintain structural homeostasis. Superimposed upon such an activation is the tendency of cells, especially in late doubling generations, to undergo heteroploidy. These heteroploid cells may not only possess an additional growth potential consistent with the proposal by the Benditts that plaques represent benign tumors deriving from mutated cells, but such cells might also develop abnormalities related to their ability to metabolize lipids. An example supporting the foregoing concept is the currently common surgical practice of replacing occluded segments of arteries by autografts of veins. The latter soon assume the structural characteristics of arteries and ultimately exhibit the stigmata of AA (Barbouriak et al., 1974).

Characteristics of the Immune Response

Thus far we have dealt with the proposal that the intimal plaque may derive from a process of clonal senescence following the activation of intimal stem cells by hemodynamic forces. In this way, the initial process in the genesis of AA can be related to aging in accordance with the Hayflick model. We have also proposed that during clonal senescence heteroploid cells emerge which may be not-self and capable of provoking an immune response. In this regard, it has been noted that there are cells with enlarged nuclei and adjacent lymphocytic infiltration, as well as cells which are coated by immunoglobulins. These observations suggest autoimmune phenomena consistent with the autoimmune theory of aging. Histopathological observations supporting these conclusions consist of areas of proliferating intimal cells with enlarged nuclei and adjacent lymphocytic infiltration; immunopathological support derives from the observation of cells coated by immunoglobulins.

In addition to the foregoing, areas of hyaline intimal thickening, with and without an infiltration of lymphocytes and histiocytes may be encountered (figures 4 and 5). Judging from the numerous illustrations in studies by Schwartz (1970), such areas often exhibit the characteristics of amyloid. The relation of amyloid to immune responses and to aging have been particularly well documented by Walford (1969). The relation of amyloid deposition to activities of the immune system is most readily comprehended when amyloidosis is associated with long-standing chronic inflammatory processes or is associated with disseminated multiple myelomatosis because of the presence of immunocytes. The association of amyloid with immune processes is less readily comprehended when amyloid occurs on a genetic basis or as an isolated or localized process without an antecedent lymphocytic or plasma cell infiltration as evidence of an underlying immune process.

Amyloid appears to have the same ultrastructural characteristics whether of genetic or immunologic origin, or even when it occurs as an isolated process. There remains, however, a considerable difference of opinion in respect to its chemical composition, especially as to whether or not it contains mucopolysaccharides. The difficulty in this regard is that amyloid evidently has a capacity for absorbing a variety of substances. However, there is also the possibility that after initial deposition amyloid may undergo a transformation or replacement by some other tissue such as collagen or hyaline. Nevertheless, there is substantial evidence that its basic core is that of an incomplete immunoglobulin (Glenner et al., 1971) with a variable amino acid sequence, and this suggests that cells of the immune system may themselves undergo clonal senescence, giving rise to deviant cells which secrete mis-specified immunoproteins.

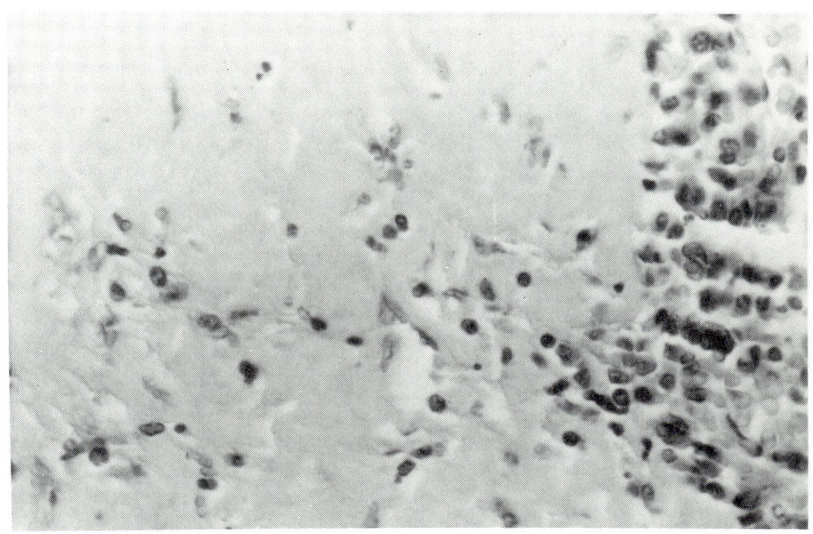

Fig. 4 Intima of aorta of 78-year-old male. H and E stain; mag. approx. 500X. Most of the area is occupied by hyaline with right border showing infiltrating lymphocytes.

An important example of a localized form of amyloidosis is that which occurs in the islets of Langerhans in diabetes. While lymphocytic infiltration of the islets has long been recognized in the juvenile form, this lesion evidently does not progress to amyloid. On the other hand, amyloid of the islets is common in the maturity-onset form without evidence of an antecedent lymphocytic infiltration. Teilum (1964) has proposed that even with an in situ formation of amyloid, the cells of origin are immunologically competent mesenchymal and reticulo-endothelial, but secrete amyloid instead of antibody when suppressed or when their antibody synthesizing function is in some way frustrated. He proposes a local deposition in a manner comparable to the laying down of collagen fibrils formed by fibroblasts.

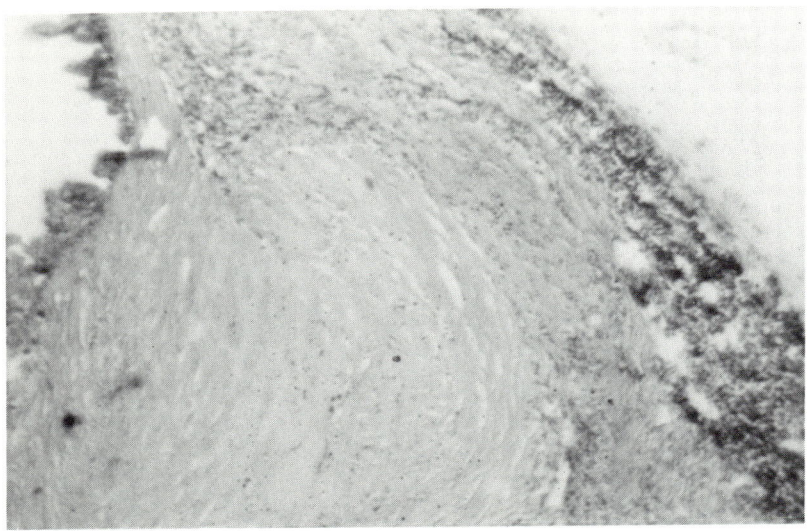

Fig. 5 Intima of aorta of 82-year-old male. H and E stain; mag. approx. 40X. Illustration shows large area of hyaline without infiltrating lymphocytes.

There is a similarity of processes between the vascular intima and the islets of Langerhans in that in both there is an antecedent appearance of presumptively heteroploid nuclei as demonstrated for islets in figure 6 and in both there is ultimately a laying down of amyloid and/or collagen (figure 7). There is a further similarity in that in both there is an associated hyperplastic or adenomatous process which may represent an aging phenomenon related to clonal senescence according to the Hayflick model.

The Origins of Lipids in Intimal Plaques

There are numerous studies which show an increase with age in plasma or serum cholesterol and triglycerides, and these have been linked with AA to account for the progressive increase with age in the incidence and severity of degenerative vascular disease. There are also many investigations dealing with the influence of the lipid content of diets, but these are not directly relevant to the aspect of the subject under discussion here. As Bierman (1973) has noted, there is also a decline with aging in the lean body mass and an increase in the proportion of adipose tissue.

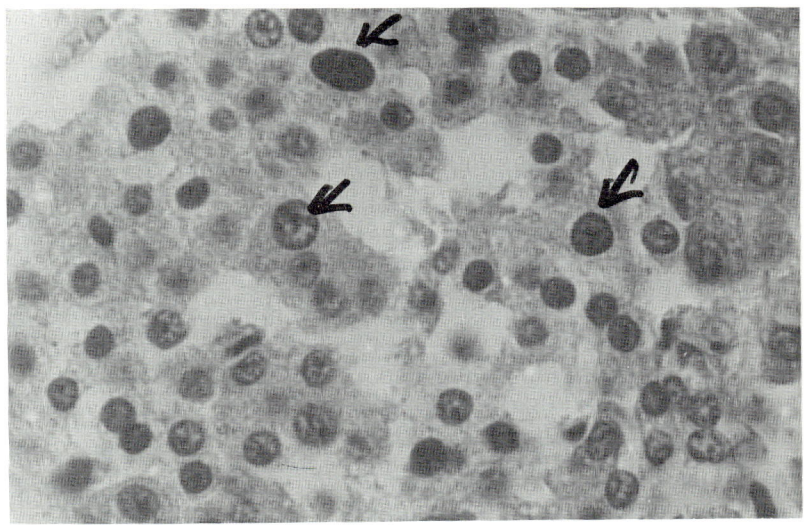

Fig. 6 Islet of Langerhans of 67-year-old diabetic female. H and E stain; mag. approx. 250X. Arrows indicate dyskaryotic cells.

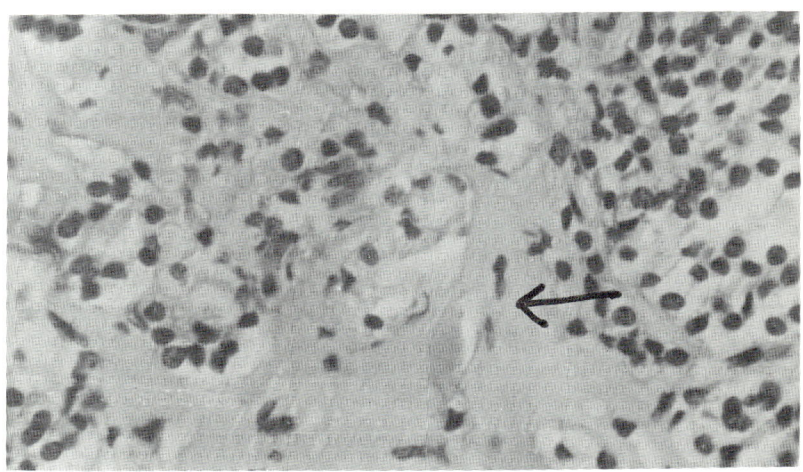

Fig. 7 Islet of Langerhans of 64-year-old diabetic female. H and E stain; mag. approx. 250X. Arrow indicates area of hyalinization.

Almost all studies dealing with lipid and body weight changes with age have been carried out in a cross-sectional design, and there are some significant parallels in respect to several of the parameters investigated. Body weight increases until a plateau is reached between 40-50 years in males and 50-60 years in females, followed by the decline noted above. Similarly, the increase with age in circulating triglyceride levels reaches a peak at 40-50 years in males and about a decade later in females, followed in each sex by a decline. Thus, the triglyceride curves are essentially superimposable on the body weight curves for adult populations. Insofar as myocardial infarction (MI) may be related to the severity of AA, there is a further parallel. In a study of 500 survivors of MI, Goldstein et al. (1973) found an overall hyperlipidemia in about one-third. However, about 50 percent of the males and almost two-thirds of the females below age 50 had either hypertriglyceridemia, hypercholesterolemia or both. On the other hand, in those over age 70 with MI (when the prevalence of MI and AA peaks) virtually no male had hyperlipidemia and only about 25 percent of females showed abnormal lipid levels.

These observations serve to point up the limitations of a cross-sectional design, since it is not possible to determine whether the decline in body weight and incidence of hyperlipidemia represents a progression in each individual or is characteristic of a genetically select group who have never been overweight or exhibited hyperlipidemia and, therefore, survived to advanced old age. There are many other curves representing functional declines with age, or changes in the incidence of disease states, which show a middle-age peak followed by a decline, and for many of these there is no evident causal link with lipid metabolism; some cancers represent a case in point. All may have common fundamental underlying cause, not yet elucidated. In any event, these observations raise doubt as to how essential hyperlipidemia is in the genesis of AA, when so many individuals with advanced AA after age 70 do not manifest this biochemical abnormality.

There is also the related question whether the hyperlipidemia is an initiating factor in AA, or simply a reflection of an intrinsic vascular tissue process. Bierman (1973) discusses the role of an intracellular lipase which is activated by a variety of peptide hormones (via cyclic AMP as a second messenger). While this enzyme has inactive as well as active forms, virtually nothing is known about its changes with age, or of any of the steps involved in the control of fatty acid metabolism. Bierman (1973) cites studies which report a lipoprotein lipase in vascular endothelium which can be displaced from its binding sites and released into the circulation by surface active heparin. Studies using this technique show a decrease with age in serum lipoprotein lipase activity. Kritchevsky and Howard (1970) have compared early and late passage cells of human fibroblasts and conclude that there is an increase in total lipid in late passage cells with the older cells showing an increase in lecithin and a decrease in phosphatides, changes which may possibly reflect alterations in cell membrane characteristics. Moreover, late passage cells remain capable of synthesizing significant amounts of cholesterol even when grown in medium devoid of exogenous lipid. Bierman concludes that aging animals as well as aging cells in tissue culture exhibit the same metabolic characteristics with regard to lipid metabolism. They synthesize less lipid, but, in general, they also metabolize less lipid.

Deficiencies of the endocrine system, and in particular those components of it which regulate carbohydrate and fat metabolism, have long been considered as influencing atherogenesis, but largely through effects on plasma lipid levels. Some observations in recent years suggest that simple substitution therapy for the hormonal deficiencies may not produce the desired ends. Thyroid hormone has been used for many years to lower hypercholesterolemia, with largely inconclusive results. There has also been considerable controversy regarding tolbutamide, a drug which enhances insulin secretion by beta cells and used in the control of maturity-onset diabetes and associated vascular sequelae (Feinstein, 1971). While this agent has had the desired effect of reducing blood glucose levels, there has been an unanticipated increase over other therapeutic measures in the incidence of MI; and there is other evidence of hyperinsulinemia associated with MI in subjects who were not diabetic prior to their heart attack (Tsabournis et al., 1968).

Some current attention has turned to investigating mechanisms at the cellular level which are influenced by hormones, and to possible aberrations in the synthesis of hormones. There are evidently changes which occur in the cytoplasmic membrane and other receptor sites of target cells of hormones, particularly in respect to adipocytes and their insulin acceptor sites (Guatrecasas, 1974). The possible alterations in cellular lipase activities in vascular tissues, as noted above, might have such an origin. There is also some investigation into possible alterations in molecular and spatial configuration of hormones. In this regard, it has been proposed that such changes in specification may occur in insulin (O'Brien et al., 1967; Blumenthal, 1968) and possibly diminish its physiological activity, as well as initiate autoimmune reactions. There is currently some interest in insulin-dependent diabetes as possibly of autoimmune origin, and the presence of amyloid in islets in maturity-onset diabetes suggests a similar possibility. It should be noted in this regard that the current extensive use of immunoassay techniques to determine circulating hormone levels may not be directly translatable to physiological activity if the reagent antibody is unable to distinguish between normal and mis-specified hormone, or if an autoantibody is present to confound the results.

In a recent study of the endocrine system (exclusive of the gonads) we have observed in all of the glands an age-related series of changes comparable to those already mentioned in respect to the islets of Langerhans as well as in cells of the vascular intima. There appears to be a progressive increase over time in the incidence of cells with dyskaryotic nuclei, of foci of adenomatous hyperplasia, of an infiltration of lymphocytes evidently targeted at the dyskaryotic cells or areas of hyperplasia, and with a diminished infiltration or absence of lymphocytes, areas of hyaline or amyloid deposition appear. Our hypothesis regarding these observations as well as the analagous observations in vascular intima is that under appropriate stimulus (in the case of the endocrine system perhaps of hypothalamic origin as suggested by Dilman (1971)), inactive or reserve cells undergo clonal proliferation in a manner analagous to the Hayflick model (adenomatous hyperplasia), in the course of which heteroploid (dyskaryotic) not-self cells appear and evoke a response of T cells of the immune system (lymphocytic infiltration). When this response diminishes, is suppressed or fails, hyaline or amyloid is deposited in the glands and autoantibodies may appear in the serum. The latter is consistent with reports of an age-related increase in the incidence of autoantibodies to several endocrine glands.

While much work remains to test this hypothesis, it could account for some of the losses in efficiency of operation of the endocrine system in relation to lipid metabolism and the genesis of AA as noted above. Two endocrine-related disorders appear to have a special relation to the initiation and intensification of AA, maturity-onset diabetes and hypothyroidism. It is generally recognized that in maturity-onset diabetes serum immunoreactive levels are normal or elevated, and it may be significant that in some cases of occlusive vascular disease hyperinsulinism is detected before the manifestations of chemical diabetes. There are also reports relating to an increased prevalence of thyroid autoantibodies in coronary AA (Bastenie et al., 1972; Heinonen et al., 1972; Fowler et al., 1973).

Conclusion

In this presentation, we have noted that subject age remains the best correlate with the incidence and severity of athero-arteriosclerosis. We have proposed a concept of the genesis of AA which relates to the Hayflick model of clonal senescence, generally considered to represent a model for biological aging at the cellular level. This model may be applied not only to alterations in intimal vascular tissues, where plaques are generated, but also to the endocrine system. In the latter, it may be associated with the development of an endocrine deficiency through a process involving the synthesis of mis-specified (not-self) hormone which may evoke an immune response, with ultimate replacement of gland parenchyma by hyaline or amyloid. Mis-specification may also occur during clonal senescence of intimal smooth muscle cells with alteration of hormone acceptor sites with resulting failure of enzymes normally involved in lipid metabolism. If this concept can be validated, AA would then qualify as a biological aging process, whether or not one chooses to make a distinction between the latter and a disease state.

REFERENCES

Adler, W. H. (1974). In "Theoretical Aspects of Aging" (M. Rockstein, M. L. Sussman, and J. Chesky, eds.), pp. 33-42, Academic Press, New York.
Anderson, T. W. (1970). The Lancet (Lond.) 2, 753.
Andres, R. (1971). Med. Clin. North America 55, 835.
Barbouriak, J. J., Pintar, K., and Korns, M. E. (1974). The Lancet (Lond.) 2, 621.
Bastenie, P. A., Bonnyns, M., Neve, P., and Vanhaelat, L. (1972). The Lancet (Lond.) 1, 1072.
Benditt, E. P., and Benditt, J. M. (1973). Proc. Nat. Acad. Sci. (USA) 70, 1753.
Bierman, E. L. (1973). Mech. Ageing Develop. 2, 315.
Blumenthal, H. T. (1967). In "Cowdry's Arteriosclerosis - A Survey of the Problem" (H. T. Blumenthal, ed.), pp. 510-528, Charles C Thomas, Springfield, Illinois.
Blumenthal, H. T. (1968). Ann. N.Y. Acad. Sci. 149, 854.
Blumenthal, H. T. (1971). Symps. Metab. and Disease, pp. 34-41, Food and Drug Directorate, Health and Welfare Ministry, Ottawa, Canada.

Blumenthal, H. T. (1972). The Gerontologist 12, 115.
Burnet, F. M. (1973). The Lancet (Lond.) 2, 480.
Burton, A. C. (1951). Am. J. Physiol. 164, 319.
Dilman, V. M. (1971). The Lancet (Lond.) 1, 1211.
Dubois, R. (1968). "So Human an Animal". Chas. Scribner's Sons, New York.
Feinstein, A. R. (1971). Clin. Pharmacol. Therap. 12, 167.
Fowler, P. B. S., Swale, J., Andrews, H., Ikram, H., and Benim, S. (1973). The Lancet (Lond.) 1, 558.
Fromm, E. (1955) "The Sane Society". Fawcett Publ. Inc., Greenwich, Connecticut.
Gelfant, S., and Grove, G. L. (1974). In "Theoretical Aspects of Aging" (M. Rockstein, M. L. Sussman, and J. Chesky, eds.), pp. 105-118, Academic Press, New York.
Glenner, G. G., Terry, W., Harada, M., Isersky, C., and Page, D. (1971). Science 172, 1150.
Goldstein, J., Hazzard, W. R., Schrott, H. G., Bierman, E. L., and Motulsky, J. (1973). J. Clin. Invest. 52, 1533.
Goldstein, S. (1974). J. Am. Med. Assoc. 230, 1651.
Goldstein, S., Niewiarowski, S., and Singal, S. P. (1975). Fed. Proc. 34, 68.
Guatrecasas, P. (1974). Hosp. Practice 9, 73.
Hayflick, L., and Moorhead, P. S. (1961). Exp. Cell Res. 25, 585.
Heinonen, O. P., Aho, K., Pyorala, K., Gordin, A., Funsar, S., and Furo, K. (1972). The Lancet (Lond.) 1, 785.
Hilleboe, H. A. (1967). In "Cowdry's Arteriosclerosis - A Survey of the Problem" (H. T. Blumenthal, ed.), p. 668, Charles C Thomas, Springfield, Illinois.
Holliday, R. (1975). Fed. Proc. 34, 51.
Kleemeier, R. W. (1965). Contemp. Psychol. 10, 53.
Kritchevsky, D., and Howard, B. V. (1970). In "Aging in Cell and Tissue Culture" (E. Holeckova and V. J. Cristofalo, eds.), pp. 57-69, Plenum Press, New York.
Long, E. R. (1967). In "Cowdry's Arteriosclerosis - A Survey of the Problem" (H. T. Blumenthal, ed.), pp. 5-20, Charles C Thomas, Springfield, Illinois.
Martin, G. M., and Sprague, C. A. (1974). Exp. Mol. Path. 13, 126.
Marx, J. L. (1975). Science 187, 526.
O'Brien, D., Shapcott, D., and Roy, C. C. (1967). Diabetes 16, 572.
Orgel, L. E. (1973). Nature (Lond.) 243, 441.
Page, I. R. (1974). Science 186, 1.
Robbins, S. L. (1974). Human Path. 5, 9.
Schwartz, P. (1970). "Amyloidosis, Cause and Manifestations of Senile Deterioration". Charles C Thomas, Springfield, Illinois.

Shock, N. W. (1974). In "Theoretical Aspects of Aging"
   (M. Rockstein, M. L. Sussman, and J. Chesky, eds.),
   pp. 119-136, Academic Press, New York.
Teilum, G. (1964). Acta Path. Microbiol. Scandinav. 61, 25.
Texon, M. (1963). In "Atherosclerosis and its Origin" (M.
   Sandler and G. H. Bourne, eds.), pp. 167-184, Academic
   Press, New York.
Tsabournis, M., Chiles, R., Ryan, J. M., and Skillman, T.
   (1968). Circulation 38, 1156.
U. S. Dept. HEW Publ. # (HSM) 72-1207. National Center for
   Health Statistics. "Health in the Later Years of Life".
   pp. 8-9.
U. S. Dept. HEW Publ. # (NIH) 72-137. "Report by NHLI Task
   Force on Arteriosclerosis". Vol. 1.
Vracko, R., and Benditt, E. P. (1974). Am. J. Path. 75, 204.
Vracko, R., and Benditt, E. P. (1975). Fed. Proc. 34, 68.
Walford, R. O. (1969). "The Immunologic Theory of Aging".
   Williams and Wilkins Co., Baltimore.
Warren, J. V. (1973). J. Chronic Diseases 26, 347.
Wilson, D. L. (1974). In "Theoretical Aspects of Aging"
   (M. Rockstein, M. L. Sussman, and J. Chesky, eds.),
   pp. 11-22, Academic Press, New York.

MEMORY AND AGING

Alvin I. Goldfarb, M. D.

7 West 96th Street
New York, New York 10025

I. INTRODUCTION

A completely exhaustive review of the topic of aging and memory is obviously beyond my capacities for a symposium presentation. However, I would like, today, to do the following: briefly define aging and discuss memory decline or impairment and their relation to each other, to clinical phenomena, and to nosology and neuropathology. I would also like to address myself to the relationship of memory and life expectancy. Finally, I would like to state my personal views on the practical medical assistance this information gives us; how views of memory decline with aging can help us set our goals and plan our care or treatment of the old and aged without excessive hopes but, yet, without undue pessimism. In this review, my primary focus will be upon permanent memory loss. I will not deal, except as they may be contributory to the irreversible states, with the transitory, acute, toxic, infectious states, conditions of poor cerebral support, specific lesions in the brain, or identifiable diseases of the central nervous system; nor will I do more than mention in passing the defects of memory with functional disorder.

II. DEFINITIONS

To me, as a physician who works in neurology and psychiatry, aging seems best defined as a decline in functional capacity; this is related to structural changes considered to be related to chronological aging either as the result of illness and accidents -- environmental insults -- or of an inevitable genetically determined life course. Some persons are truly aged because of illness and accidents, others for genetically determined reasons; the two are usually intertwined.

It is difficult or impossible to separate inevitable,

genetically determined aging from the effects of those processes we call diseases, because they are referable to definable assaultive agents from within or without the organism or due to acquired or inborn metabolic errors. At any rate, with aging the individual becomes increasingly vulnerable to death from any cause; there is an increasing vulnerability to strain from stress. The structurally based functional changes responsible do not occur at the same speed in all individuals or in all organs or systems of the individual. Unfortunately, caretakers of old persons tend to talk loosely and when the decline in functional capacity is of systems such as the skeletal, urogenital, pulmonary, gastrointestinal or cardiovascular, the incapacity is often regarded as infirmity, impairment or debility and the person is called old, frail, infirm or handicapped, but when the decline is in remembering and being able to use one's mind, then the individual is called senile. Also, that the disorder of mentation may be directly referable to the loss of brain tissue is sometimes overemphasized and at other times forgotten; all too often memory loss of the old is ascribed to social and psychological "causes" and treatment is mistakenly and often psychonoxiously directed.

Memory, or remembering, can be defined as a change in the organism's interaction with previously experienced environmental challenges when these are re-presented in whole, part or by symbol. It is a use of the past, as experienced as in some sense organismically recorded, for present purposes. Whether it is a trace and whether this is molecular, cellular, intracellular or intersynaptic, an alteration in a complex field of forces, localized or non-localized but patterned, is beyond my capacity for discussion.

The importance of memory is obvious; it is that aspect of adaptation that makes us sentient, responsive, interactional. Consciousness itself is most likely simply an awareness of being aware and therefore a memory, a recognition that one has responded; it is a response to a response. Without postulation of an homonculus, consciousness may be likened to the self-viewing itself because of the self's possession of a "TV" or cinematic time machine which views the self's action of a millisecond before, while continuing in the action which it therefore becomes capable of modifying. This could be couched in neurologic terms analogous to those which describe cerebellar coordination of motor acts. From this point of view, in psychological terms, memories are the conscious mental events that follow and influence homeostasis and the interaction between individuals and the environment by means of the receptors, effectors, and central nervous system. What we call memory may be the only conscious mental events that accompany, or rather immediately follow, and thus become a part of this interplay. Loss of memory constitutes a loss in consciousness and of psychological and social self; if large enough, it leads to the loss of life. It does so not only by interfering with the individual's capacity to deal adequately with current events and to meet the challenges of the changing world and to maintain homeostasis, but also, from the human point of view, even before biologic death, by converting the self-conscious person into a vegetative organism.

In practice, in psychological theory, or on neuroanatomical or neuropathological grounds, it is not possible to separate memory from learning; *i.e.*, one remembers what one has learned, can remember what one learns, learning is measured by what one remembers. We depend upon memory for the simplest adaptive behavior and survive complex challenges to integrity by having learned and by remembering. There are, of course, many kinds of learning which relate to a number of types of memory; habituation results in remembering what need not be attended to, sensitization does the opposite, conditioning of inhibitory, associative or reinforcement type yields memories that lead to avoidance, flow of ideas, or to approach and specific action. Much of what is learned and leads to altered action, especially if it is visceral and occurs with little or no responsive awareness, does not lead to what we generally speak about as memory or remembering (Razran, 1971). We generally talk about memory, or remembering, within the context of so-called consciousness; therefore, my remarks will be directed almost exclusively toward the type of remembering that becomes part of, or constitutes, conscious thought.

Learning, whether of seeming, primary importance and intended or essential, or simply incidental and subject to useless and unexpected recall, requires, first, registration, impression or recording. Second, information is held, stored, cycled, rehearsed for a variable period of time; there is a reverberant kind of remembering even while other registrations are occurring, as in the lingering of musical notes while new ones fall on the ear. Third, there is storage -- a holding for a longer time, perhaps the lifetime of the individual or of that tissue or cells which make such "holding" possible. Such "storage" or holding may be conceived of as a static and geographic change, or as a process in one or more possibly shifting locales. The storage can be attributed to changes in molecular, chemical or structural patterning or to the persistence, or the potential for the recreation of, fields of force.

The three arbitrarily heuristically described steps are followed by a second series; it is these which are usually recognized or referred to as remembering. They are, first -- recall, remembering, finding or retrieving; second -- recognition of the remembrance as "correct", and third -- utilization. Utilization may be by way of overt verbalization or action of a mental or physical type, or it may be implicit and part of the process called thought whether or not the thought be a part of awareness. As previously mentioned in this discussion, we must probably be limited to that remembering which remains in or can be revived to awareness.

The efficiency of such processes which are called learning or memory, depending on whether we place emphasis on the first three or the last three steps, appears to decrease with increasing age in years. This is true whether learning is measured in terms of its speed, or by the amount recalled or recognized or utilized. However, if ample time is given for registration, for reinforcing short term holding or rehearsal, and for coding or categorizing of information, as well as for its assimilation and "storage", many old persons may do as well as most young persons. This may be true even when no extra time is given for recall, recognition or utilization.

Memory loss is a decrease in the capacity to remember responses based upon prior experience and to learn or re-learn responses useful in the continuing sequence of adjustments necessary for adaptation. Memory loss may be true (*i.e.*, actual) or spurious. True memory loss appears to be inextricably interwoven with true biological aging -- that is, with tissue loss or change. It is this decline in mental functioning that is usually called senility; this loss appears to be related to a decrease in adaptive and survival capacity. Spurious memory loss -- a feeling or conviction that memory is poor, although objectively this cannot be established -- is commonly present in depressed and anxious older persons.

I cannot do justice here to the large problem of what may be considered normal or average changes in memory with aging. Psychological investigative reports on such matters are prolix, inconclusive, and peppered with confusing terminology. It is possible, however, to make some generalizations from these reports, from everyday observation and from work with a variety of old patients whose chief complaint is not defective memory. These general statements are made as a bridge to the consideration of the conditions in which memory loss is a chief complaint and is associated with changes in the origin of the mind, the brain.

III. NORMAL SENESCENT MEMORY LOSS

An example of the difficulty in assessing what "normally" happens to memory with aging is the observation by Botwinick (1967) that, in surviving males, memory declines less than in females after the age of 80. This may well be because those who survive are the relatively stalwart; males of lesser strengths and ability -- including memory -- have died off by then. The lower female death rate at all ages may serve to defer the demise of the old female with poor memory. The need for, and the difficulty of obtaining longitudinal data, is obvious and the perils of generalization from cohort studies are many.

It is tempting to ascribe decline of memory in aging to "normal", average, inevitable losses that must occur at genetically determined different rates in individuals of the species and is therefore displayed in varying degrees by persons who "live to a ripe old age". A few persons could be expected to survive, because of unusual health of other systems than the central nervous, to a very old age, at which time the brain changes would be increasingly revealed. This is an idea advanced by Jonathan Swift in his descriptions of the Struldbrugs encountered by Gulliver in his travels.

It now seems more likely that the normal decline in mental functional capacity does not yield a progression to the point of recognizable senility unless there are specific accelerants to the loss of functioning brain. The process may be accelerated first by the advent of illness and physical impairment which damages or leads to poor support of the brain or, second, by as yet unidentified factors which lead to cerebral cortical cell loss with greater rapidity than normally occurs in the presence of otherwise seemingly good physical health. Among the first are febrile states, uremia, electrolyte imbalance, anoxia and hypoxia for whatever reason, hypoglycemia, hypertension or hypotension -- conditions which occur with diseases, accidents and malnutrition. In the second group "causes" are as yet unknown; heredity appears to be important, latent viruses may play a role and other factors may, retrospectively, be viewed as having been so obvious as to defy identification.

However this may be, other factors being equal, it seems that persons of higher social class, as measured by years of education and occupation have better memories in old age than those of less education and lower occupational status. This appears to be true for the "normal" (Birren, 1964; Botwinick, 1967; Jarvick and Cohen, 1973) and also for the old with mental impairment (Goldfarb, 1960). Such social class -- or educational and occupational -- determined sparing of memory or increase in vulnerability to loss acts to mask or accentuate memory decline and to obstruct the devising of a single valid measure of impairment for all old persons.

Not only do socioeconomic factors influence memory with aging, but the brighter the person in early life the better memory holds up in later life. Again, this may have genetic determinants; but without question genetic potential is influenced by nurture. Such individual differences add their difficulty in the measure of memory loss.

Also, persons who continue in work or who have equivalent activities have better memories in chronologic old age than those who do not. Such a relationship appears to stem from the early interactions of nature and nurture referred to but may illustrate the continued influence of activity upon memory and of learning upon activity. It is a special instance of "them as has gits, while them as hasn't, loses". The aged who have learned to learn and how to do it, in whom there is expectancy and set for learning undoubtedly learn more and remember more -- unless there supervenes a defect of retrieval and use -- than the old who are not similarly self-directed, motivated and skilled. Furthermore, the higher the genetic endowment, the more likely the development of these attributes and the greater the possibility of favorable socioeconomic conditions because of the "selection of parents".

Possibly related to changes in motivation, attention, concentration or to changes in the sensory-neural-perceptual apparatus and its organization is the observation that in old persons retention of auditory material appears to be better, generally, than visual (Arenberg, 1967). It is likely that many such differences evolve in the aging person whose sensory receptors change with time and whose central nervous system may become altered in its redundancy, complexity and flexibility.

With aging, more complex material is forgotten more quickly than the simple matters; complexity, however, depends upon the capacities and past training of the individual. Secretaries, professionals, laborers, housewives, perform quite differently with respect to memory and learning.

This is, of course, in line with the fact that past skills contribute to relearning and to new learning even at advanced age. There are savings, whatever has been forgotten, interfered with or decayed. Just as complex motor acts involved in skating, swimming, bicycling and driving can be revived more quickly than they can be newly learned, and just as there may be transfer from one skill of this type to another, there are savings and transfers in the more implicit and more symbolically constituted aspects of behavior. There seems little question, from everyday observation, that in the highly verbal aspects of behavior the prior organization and assimilation by way of coding and categorizing contributes to the endurance of memories or their facile revival in that "structure" and theoretical concepts facilitate remembering.

Thus, the complex interrelationship of memories contributes to their continuance. Furthermore, what has been reinforced, relearned or has become habit remains longest. There is a highly protective value to the automatization of adaptively useful skills, information, habits, and ways of life of physical, emotional, psychological and social type. The more one learns and the more one has learned, the greater the likelihood one will be able to learn even in old age. There are, however, somatic changes with growing old that may be, in our present state of knowledge, unavoidable.

It is likely that a mild to moderate decline in the capacity to remember with chronologic aging is related to the brain cell loss in persons regarded as normal, average and in good physical health. The decline does not, however, assume grand proportions and although they may be subjectively troublesome and objectively discernible, they are tolerable to the self and to society. Usually, except in special situations and for special types of occupation or performance, the memory loss is not incompatible with continuation of a normal life. This normal decline may be related to a loss of cortical neurones with chronologic aging. According to Brody (1973) there is, by age 55 years, a reduction in cortical neurones of about 25%; by age 80 about 25% more are lost; only about 5/8 of the original cell population have survived (figure 1).

Similarly, data compiled by Weil (1945) (Table I) from various sources shows that the weight of the brain falls about five percent from young adulthood to the beginning of the ninth decade. This decrease in brain weight may well be on the basis of loss of cortical neurones.

These data on cerebral cell loss and decrease in brain weight in persons presumably competent at death suggests that a surprisingly large cortical neurone cell loss is well tolerated and that a cortical cell loss under 50% and brain weight decrease of less than 5 to 8% is consistent with normal function. As one moves to greater cell loss, memory obviously suffers. This is what is referred to as the senile state. The clinical and neuropathological aspects of these greater cell losses and decreases in brain weight will be briefly discussed.

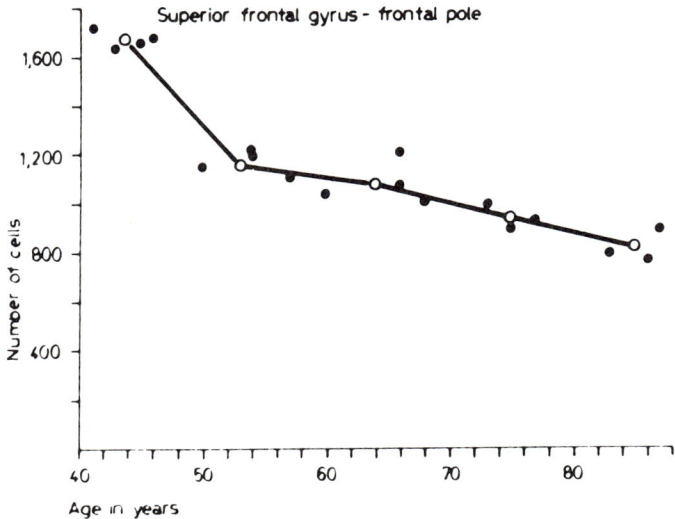

Fig. 1 The relationship of age to cell number in the superior frontal gyrus (from Brody, 1973).

Table I

Weight of Brain in Relation to Age, Sex, and Stature*

Age in Years	Weight in Grams		
	Males		Females
	Cerebrum	Total Brain	Total Brain
1-2		1105	995
3-6		1170	1100
7-13		1400	1165
14-19		1360	1240
20-29	1200	1365	1250
30-39	1180	1350	1230
40-49	1170	1310	1220
50-59	1120	1320	1270
60-69	1140	1320	1200
70-79	1150	1305	1140

*Figures calculated as mean values from data on English brains published by Pearl for the cerebrum and by Gladstone for the total brain (Biometrika 4, 104, 148, 1905) (from Weil, 1945).

IV. SENILE MEMORY LOSS

So far I have discussed what is generally spoken about as normal or senescent decline. There is a large qualitative difference between such changes and the senile state. A large loss of the capacity for remembering, whether or not this is understood and reacted to by the afflicted individual, is catastrophic if permanent. Memory loss of relatively severe degree may be transient or permanent depending upon whether brain cells are rendered dysfunctional or are killed by somato-pathologic states; memory loss may be transient on the basis of emotional or psychological causes, the pathophysiology of which still defies understanding. Before considering the losses of memory that are truly associated with aging, memory loss of a "non-organic" type must be touched upon.

Functional Transient Memory Loss

In senescence, as in youth, memory loss is seen in depressive and elated states and in disorders of thought content like the paranoid states. These may be mistaken for senile changes. In these "functional disorders", attention and concentration may be poor, there may be preoccupation, distractibility, poor motivation, and lack of cooperation with examiners. There is often, in depressed persons, a subjective experience of poor memory which usually cannot be objectively confirmed; memory may, by some tests of performance, be poorer than in the past. When the episode of illness is over, the subjective sense of poor memory leaves and objective performance improves. In paranoid states, complaints about memory usually cannot be objectively confirmed but, if the patient has received electroconvulsant treatment -- a cause of normally transient amnesia -- complaints may persist. Also, the functional disorders may complicate or be complicated by any of the other memory disorders. This is a frequent cause of clinical confusion and can lead to mistakes in prognosis and treatment. Because treatment itself may lead to potentially reversible memory defects, the initial state of the patient should be properly evaluated.

Electroconvulsant treatment of functional mental disorders usually leads to transient memory loss. The amount and duration of the loss is usually related to the number and frequency of treatments given, but is usually reversed with return of remembering after periods of a few weeks to several months. In old persons, some memory defects may persist for a year or more and, again, such memory loss may merge into defects of memory occurring for reasons mentioned above. In the course of electroshock treatment, petit mal attacks not followed by an induced grand mal seizure will result in an especially severe degree of memory loss for a period of hours or days. Also, drug treatment of the functional mental disorders can be a cause of what has been referred to as acute brain syndrome by direct pharmacological action on the brain or by way of cardiovascular effects.

Organic Memory Loss: The Acute, Reversible Disorders

Relatively severe degrees of memory loss occur as part of a large number of clinical conditions in old persons. These are subdivisible into two major groups. The first includes the disorders of memory that are potentially reversible in whole or in part, and are therefore transient unless the underlying disorder leads to death or the condition is permitted to persist so long that memory loss becomes permanent. These transient conditions can be ascribed to cellular dysfunction under circumstances of poor cerebral support or intoxication by drugs or metabolites. Among the most common reasons for poor cerebral support are trauma and cerebral edema or hemmorhage, cardiac, pulmonary or renal malfunction, hyper- and hypoglycemia, electrolyte imbalance, polycythemia, anemia, malnutrition, anoxia, infection, drug intoxication, and specific avitaminosis, and endocrine dyscrasias. Similarly, cerebrovascular emboli, thrombi or spasm, by interfering with circulation, may be initiating incidents. Such conditions result in what is called acute organic brain syndrome. "Acute" indicates that the dysfunction of cerebral neuronal elements can be reversed by improvement in the pathophysiology and that the state is transitory. It must be emphasized that many of these acute conditions may be "chronically present" unless recognized and corrected. As in the case of mild chronic cardiac failure, hypotension, avitaminosis, and endocrine disease, potentially reversible memory loss can merge into and become irreversible if these disorders persist over a long period. If the cerebrum is severely deprived suddenly and intensely for a short period, or to a lesser degree for long periods, cells are irreversibly damaged. When the number of cells destroyed reaches a threshold for the person, the result is residual permanent defect. Because recovery is often slow, the extent of the defect that is irreversible may not be certain for some months. In old persons, for example, episodes of low blood pressure which may occur with surgical operation and anesthesia, or following a fracture or myocardial infarction, may yield an episode of severe memory loss which contributes to, or accentuates and possibly first brings to attention, a loss of memory which was previously present and was possibly progressing.

Transient memory loss may be closely related to center-encephalic dysfunction. For example, dysfunction in the hippocampal areas of the temporal lobes, the mammillary bodies, in the regions surrounding the 3rd and 4th ventricles, and in the medial nuclei of the hypothalamus appears to occur under circumstances of prolonged thiamin deficiency. When such cell dysfunction or damage occurs, it may be accompanied by or contribute to changes in the cortex of the brain. As mentioned, nutritional correction may correct or greatly improve the patient's status, but if too many cells have already died then memory loss, which initially appeared to be chiefly for more immediate matters and recent events, becomes permanent and the extent of remote memory loss is noted to be greater and apparently progressive.

Senile Memory Loss: The Permanent, Chronic Impairments

The second large group, the permanent, chronic disorders, has been alluded to in description of the acute or transitory conditions. Permanent memory losses can occur because of trauma, intoxication or the failure of nutritive and metabolic supports to the brain. But, in addition, there are losses of cells that appear to be related to a genetically determined life span of the postmitotic cerebral cortical neurones. It is possible that what is presumed to be genetically determined actually may be the effects of as yet unknown destructive factors upon the cortex of the brain and to the limbic system. If genetic in origin, there may well be more than one type of inheritance; in some there may be programming of the probable life of the cells under any conditions; in others there may be increased vulnerability to common or unusual environmental insults of infectious or noninfectious type. Also, the disorders may be genetically multifactorial with highly differing degrees of certainty of emergence under varying conditions. It is these disorders that have been recognized and referred to as the senile dementias and the presenile dementias; the term "Alzheimer's Disease" may be most felicitously applied to both for neuropathological reasons discussed below. It is important to note that these "senile brain changes" may be added to the effects of or be joined by the cell losses incurred because of trauma, infection, general disease and focal damages.

V. NEUROPATHOLOGY AND PATHOPHYSIOLOGY

A complete, organized discussion of neuropathology and pathogenesis exceeds the scope of this paper. Despite popular opinion, both lay and medical, to the contrary, intracranial cerebral athero- or arteriosclerosis is not an important primary cause of memory loss, nor is the extracerebral narrowing of internal carotid or vertebral arteries that may result in episodes of transient ischemia and lead to stroke. Adams (1974), based on his observations and those of Barr (1955) and Lassen (1961), states: "Belief in senility conditioned by faulty cerebral plumbing dies hard, but there is no pathological or physiological evidence to support the theory that widespread degeneration of nerve cells and tracts found in dementia in old age results from ischemia caused by atheromatosis. Indeed, it seems more likely that parenchymatous degeneration in the grey matter comes first; reduced oxygen, tension and blood flow follow in a diffuse, slowly progressive process in which atheroma and anoxia play no part." These sentiments are apparently shared and confirmed by numerous other investigators.

General memory loss is a reflection of decreased neuronal number or mass. The decrease in brain weight and the neuronal loss described by Brody (1973) and Weil (1945) may represent relatively normal decrements reflected by little or no important memory loss. They possibly may be correlated with the slowing of learning and the capricious, or slightly impaired for detail, memory of the non-demented old. It is not normal, however, to be a dotard, to have memory losses which interfere with performance of necessary activities of daily life, and it is these persons in whom cortical atrophy and dilated ventricles are found. The degree of atrophy and the subsequent dilation of at least the lateral ventricles appears to be proportional to the clinically measurable amount of memory loss, although mild to moderate degrees of loss may be socially unobserved.

Goldfarb and Jahn (1959), from Rothschild's data (1937, 1942), postulated that a loss in brain weight of about 6% was associated with clinically mild to moderate memory loss, over 12% with at least moderate memory loss, and that a 20% decrease in brain weight was concordant with severe memory defects (Table II). This is in agreement with the report of Kiev *et al.* (1962) that a 10 to 15% brain weight loss is accompanied by clinically recognizable dementia. Even in persons with such a relatively high degree of memory loss, cerebral athero- or arteriosclerosis is not routinely found and, conversely, vascular pathology can be present with no

Table II

The Expected Relation of Selected Characteristics With
Intellectual Defect in the Chronologically Old*

Characteristic	Degree of Defect				
Intellectual deficit, clinical	None to minimal	Minimal to mild	Mild to moderate	Moderate to severe	Severe
1. Mental status questionnaire: no. of errors	0	0-2	3-5	6-8	9+
2. Face-hand test errors:					
eyes closed	0	0	0-2	2-4	4
eyes open	0	0	0	1-3	4
3. Activities of daily life (self-sufficiency)	Good	Good	Fair	Poor	Very poor
4. Mood disturbance	0-4+	0-4+	0-3+	0-4+	0
5. Thinking disorder	0-4+	0-4+	0-2+	0-4+	0
6. Overt behavior disorder	0-4+	0-4+	1+-4+	2+-4+	2+-4+
7. Incontinence:					
bladder	0	0	0-1+	0-2+	1+-4+
bowel	0	0	0	0-2+	1+-4+
8. Electroencephalogram: Amount of slow waves	Normal	Normal to minimal abnormality	Normal to minimal abnormality	Diffuse abnormality	Normal or diffuse abnormality
9. Ventricular size echoencephalography (angiogram or P.E.G.)	Normal	Normal	Moderate dilatation	Moderate to considerable increase	Great enlargement
10. Air over cortex (P.E.G.)	None	None	Slight amount	Slight to considerable amount	Slight to considerable amount
11. Average brain weight, grams	1300	1221	1220	1153	1025
12. O_2 utilization	Normal	Normal	Normal to slight decrease	Decreased	Decreased
13. Blood flow	Normal	Normal	Normal to slight decrease	Decreased	Decreased
14. Life expectancy (for age)	Normal	Normal	Normal	Usually decreased	Decreased

*From Goldfarb, 1973.

loss of memory. Vascular pathology, when it is present, appears to be merely contributory to the cell losses and is neither sufficient nor necessary for the clinical state of memory loss.

Willanger et al. (1968), from a study investigating the relationship of intellectual impairment to encephalography, concluded that psychological testing can predict radiologic demonstration of cerebral atrophy. Working with Dr. S. Antin of the neuroradiology department at Mt. Sinai Hospital, New York, I have found that our tests of memory (Tables III, IV and V) -- especially the "Mental Status Questionnaire" (M.S.Q.) described below -- are similarly predictive of cortical atrophy and ventricular dilatation as demonstrable by angiography or pneumo-encephalography (Goldfarb and Antin, 1974).

Table III

Mental Status Questionnaire - "Special 10"*

Question	Presumed test area
1. Where are we now?	Place - learning
2. Where is this place (located)?	Place - learning
3. What is today's date- day of month?	Time - learning
4. What month is it?	Time - learning
5. What year is it?	Time - learning
6. How old are you?	Memory-recent or remote
7. What is your birthday?	Memory-recent or remote
8. What year were you born?	Memory - remote
9. Who is president of the U.S.?	General information - memory
10. Who was president before him?	General information - memory

*As modified from Goldfarb, 1964b.

Table IV

Rating of Mental Functional Impairment by Mental Status Questionnaire*

No. of errors	Presumed mental status
0-2	Chronic brain syndrome absent or mild
3-8	Chronic brain syndrome moderate
9-10	Chronic brain syndrome severe
Nontestable	Chronic brain syndrome severe#

*As modified from Goldfarb, 1964b.
#In the not uncooperative person without deafness or insuperable language barrier.

Table V

Order of Stimulation Used in Face-Hand Test*

1. Right cheek-left hand 2. Left cheek-right hand 3. Right cheek-right hand 4. Left cheek-left hand	Initial trials. Response evaluated in context of further trials.
5. Right cheek-left cheek 6. Right hand-left hand	Teaching trials. Almost always correctly reported. Examiner informs or reinforces response that there were two touches.
7. Right cheek-left hand 8. Left cheek-right hand 9. Right cheek-right hand 10. Left cheek-left hand	Incorrect response and stimulation not reported, felt but displaced, projected or located in space is presumptive of brain damage.

*As modified from Goldfarb, 1964b.

Memory impairment and cerebral atrophy are very highly correlated in Willanger's series of 300 cases, more so for cortical than for ventricular dilatation, and was closest for the combination of the two. In my own smaller number of cases, ventricular dilatation alone is closely related to the mental status questionnaire score. They agree that a reduction in brain weight of about 6 to 7% appears to occur normally from the 2nd to the 7th decade of life and is not radiologically determinable. Their radiologic studies demonstrate that the decrease in size with mental impairment suggests far greater weight loss than in the normal, is radiologically discernible, and that atrophy with aging is not normal. Thus, memory defect is closely related to the decrease in brain weight as suggested by brain size, as measured by radiology. Also, Willanger et al. (1968) found that increasing chronologic age in their series appeared to "accelerate the effect" of cerebral disorder on mental impairment: older persons were more impaired than young persons with equivalent amounts of atrophy. They were unable to demonstrate that stroke or cerebral arteriosclerosis yields atrophy or dementia, but were able to demonstrate that decline in the ability to remember and cerebral atrophy go hand in hand. Similarly, Antin and I found no vascular abnormalities in our series of patients with memory loss, only dilated ventricles and cortical atrophy (Goldfarb and Antin, 1974).

Worm-Petersen and Pakkenberg (1968) state "....the occurrence of.... dementia was examined in 108 patients, all of whom presented moderate to severe atherosclerosis in the basal cerebral vessels at autopsy. One-half of the brains originated from patients who died in a hospital, the other half from patients who underwent medico-legal autopsy because of sudden, unexpected, or violent death. The majority of the cases showed signs of dementia only if pathological processes were present in the parenchyma of the brain at the same time; thus atherosclerosis in the basal vessels of the brain does not appear by itself to play any decisive role in the manifestation of dementia in old age." It is their opinion that "on the basis of the literature and our investigations that the clinical diagnosis, cerebral arteriosclerosis, is inappropriate for use in the neurologic clinic. The diagnosis has the air of being an etiological and pathogenic diagnosis, and neither of these is completely correct. We suggest that the diffuse, clinical symptoms of age, without definite etiology, should be grouped under the diagnosis 'senile encephalopathy'."

It should be added that, as in Rothschild's data (1937) and that of Corsellis (1962), atherosclerosis of smaller vessels is of no more than contributory importance in the evolution of memory loss; such changes may be present in the absence of dementia and of no great degree where dementia is severe (Corsellis, 1962; Simon and Malamud, 1965).

Thus, it now seems quite certain that it is diffuse, widespread cortical damage in the central nervous system, not usually vascular in pathogenesis, that interferes with learning and memory in a general way. The constant accompaniment of clinically important memory loss is cortical atrophy, with loss of cortical and other neurones that can be observed as a decrease in brain size and weight. The diffuse damage finally seen, however, may be preceded or accompanied by a loss of cells in the hippocampi, mammillary bodies and medial nuclei of the thalamus (Fisher and Adams, 1964; Adams et al., 1965; DeJong et al., 1969; Victor et al., 1971). By contrast, general memory loss is not necessarily a concomitant of focal damage to the various areas of the central nervous system which can nevertheless interfere with specific sensory-neural perceptive processes necessary for the recall, recognition and utilization of many specific aspects of memory to yield aphasias, apraxias and agnosias.

Cortical atrophy and ventricular dilatation are pathognomonic of an irreversible state of memory loss, but the cortical atrophy is not always easily demonstrable by radiographic techniques in the permanent form; also, with acute, reversible memory loss ventricular dilatation and cortical atrophy may be mild or absent. Recently, there has been a relative furor about the possible reversibility of dementia by recognition of ventricular dilatation based upon diminished arachnoid villi resorptive powers and a resultant normal pressure hydrocephalus. In such conditions, air over the cortex by pneumo-encephalogram is not demonstrable, at least in many cases, it has been claimed. This type of hydrocephalus is seen in younger persons who have suffered subarachnoid hemorrhages or with meningitis, and is usually self-resolving. The degree of residual memory loss in persons who have suffered this condition is not well documented. This condition appears to be actually of little or no importance in the old. The radiographic diagnostic criteria for this "syndrome" -- dementia, ataxia and incontinence -- in the old were at first presented with precision but are now unclear and imprecise. Furthermore, the concurrence of dementia, ataxia and incontinence in the old is common and of multiple and varied etiology. It is therefore no surprise that widespread use of ventricular shunts of several kinds has not yielded good results, and there is no indication that these operations are of value in the correction of memory loss in old age.

The medically popular ascription of permanent memory loss in the chronologically old to atherosclerosis carries with it the implication that it is reduced cerebral circulation and decreased oxygen supply to the brain that results in its cell losses or deterioration. This harks back to Geschichter's view (1959) that aging is the result of cardiovascular failure to support organic demands and requirements. It is true that emboli, thromboses and, very likely vasospasm, cause local tissue ischemia and infarction. Such damage to the brain is often accompanied by diffuse cerebral edema which compromises cells in distant parts. Thus, shortly after an episode of ischemia and infarction there may be generalized neuronal dysfunction reflected by an acute organic brain syndrome, acute in the sense that it subsides in entirety or in largest part. There may be residual focal signs and, also, the local tissue loss may add to pre-existing cortical cell loss. The cortical cell losses, added to those already present, may contribute to the emergence of a permanent memory loss as a concomitant of whatever organic mental state -- agnosia, apraxia, aphasia -- also emerges.

That cerebral athero- or arteriosclerosis alone, however, is not the important single cause of relatively severe diffuse cortical cerebral damage is also shown by longitudinal studies (Goldfarb, 1965). It was found in the survivors of over 1700 institutionalized persons examined yearly that the diagnosis of patients with memory loss tends to change as they age from "cerebral arteriosclerosis" to "senile dementia". Observation revealed that the patients who changed little over the years, did so slowly and gradually, although in some there might have been an acceleration of the disorder because of episodes of acute illness. In many cases, the diagnosis of cerebral arteriosclerosis may be made because a stroke called attention to an already marginally competent patient. A clearer illustration that cerebral athero- or arteriosclerosis is overly used as an explanation of memory loss is the observation of Willanger (Willanger et al., 1968) that "the majority of patients who suffer from apoplexy have normal working capacity until their first stroke, and after the stroke do not show any evidence of chronic lack of cerebral oxygen". To this may be added that many persons post-stroke can resume work and show no serious memory losses.

Kety (1960) has shown that with senile dementia, brain oxygen utilization is decreased (Table VI). It is likely that decreased brain call for oxygen and blood are indicators of, rather than explanations for, tissue loss: they denote brain cell death.

Table VI

Cerebral Oxygen Consumption and Mental State*

Condition	Cerebral oxygen consumption (% of normal)
Senile psychosis	82
Diabetic acidosis	82
Insulin hypoglycemia	79
Artificial hypothermia	67
Surgical anesthesia	64
Insulin coma	58
Diabetic coma	52
Alcoholic coma	49
Normal sleep	97
Schizophrenia	100
LSD psychosis	101
Mental arithmetic	102
Anxiety	118
Epinephrine infusion	122

*From Kety, 1960.

In the "normal" old person, learning and attempts to remember cause desynchronization of the electroencephalogram (EEG) with increase in frequency. In the old person with memory loss, the EEG may show a high amount of slow waves at rest and failure of desynchronization to take place when the individual is challenged by stimuli. Jahn (personal communication, 1975), working at the New York Medical College, suggests that computer analysis of systematically-plotted evoked potentials may provide much early information about memory loss. With challenge there may be no increase in oxygen utilization and no increase in cerebral circulation; all this may indicate either failure to respond on the basis of non-testability because of no rapport or that brain tissue is dead; the cells are non-functional.

Macroscopic decrease in brain weight, cortical atrophy and ventricular dilatation are the concomitants of permanent memory deficit. Microscopically, in all states of permanent memory loss, there is found a decrease in neuronal cell count, an abundance of amyloid plaques, neurofibrillary degeneration, granulovacuolar degeneration and deposition of lipofuscin in cell cytoplasm. The electron microscope reveals, in most but not all types, twisting of axon microtubules. This microscopic picture is the final common end of what may be a number of deteriorative or assaultive processes. Microvascular changes may be present in variable degrees not concordant with the degree of impairment.

Blessed, Thomlinson and Roth (Roth et al., 1966; Blessed et al., 1968; Roth, 1971) have shown that there is a close relationship between the number of amyloid plaques found at autopsy and the degree of dementia. Their counts suggest that no separation can be made between so-called presenile and senile states. They state, "the difference between grossly demented, mildly demented, and well preserved old people may well lie in a different progression of one and the same process assessed, albeit crudely, by plaque counts." Their findings suggest that the cell loss with chronologic aging results in, or from, amyloid plaque formation and that the number of plaques is concordant with the intensity of the accompanying intellectual deterioration, except that in so-called presenile and senile dementia the plaque counts, while high, are more variable. This suggests that the "presenile and senile dementias" do differ qualitatively from other types of senile changes in the brain. They too agree that vascular pathology has been overemphasized in the past: "in the presence of senile degenerative change the effect of cerebral transient ischemia tends to be potentiated. It seems likely also that if attention is concentrated on isolated episodes or symptoms, arteriosclerotic psychosis is likely to be diagnosed to excess."

There remains a lack of clarity about whether the Alzheimer type of brain change and severe memory loss is inevitable in persons without a genetic diathesis if only they should live long enough. Can infections, trauma, metabolic and cerebral nonsupportive processes lead to the Alzheimer type changes?

There is strong suggestion that sudden, intense cerebral deprivation of oxygen as with shock and immersion, may yield significant measurable cell loss with varying degrees of memory loss. Also, an accumulation of insults over a period of time may accelerate normal brain cell loss. But it is probable that one or more special disorders of inherited type (Lassen, 1961; Sjögren et al., 1952) are responsible for severe memory loss of old age uncomplicated by focal signs. Lauter and Meyer (1968) believe the presenile and senile disorders to be "one disease entity with different ages of manifestation". They believe this state to be unrelated to either normal aging or cerebral arteriosclerosis. They state, "neuropathologically there is a large group in which senile and arteriosclerotic changes occur together. Whether these mixed anatomical findings are relevant for the clinical symptomatology is an open question. The results of psychological investigations disagree with the usual assumption that senile dementia is only an accelerated and intensified 'senile involution'." It seems that memory loss is related to the amount of diffuse cortical neuronal loss and focal signs, when present, to cerebral arteriosclerosis.

While cortical cell losses seem sufficient on a structural basis to explain memory loss, there are also usually extensive changes also present in the limbic area. At times these may exceed those in the cortex. It may be that these are the initial changes related to loss of memory and that they remain of enduring importance when memory loss becomes permanent.

In clinical practice it is clear that, while loss of remembering (by our crude clinical measures) is grossly concordant with decreased brain weight and neuronal loss, there are nevertheless differences in individual reaction displayed with such losses. These differences can be explained on the basis of the individual's prior establishment of physical, emotional, psychological and social patterns as suggested in Table VII. Differences in reaction type because of these variations may lead to classification which incorrectly ascribes behavior to brain changes.

Table VII

The Presumptive Relationship of Etiologic Factors to Acquired Intellectual Deficit and Associated "Functional" Disorders in the Aged*

Multiple Etiology →	Brain Disturbance →	Manifestations →	Psychiatric Syndrome
Early and late physical factors: genetic accidents illness poisons	Cerebral malsupport (reversible=acute) Cerebral damage (irreversible=chronic)	Disorientation of time place person situation Memory loss recent remote Decrease in general information and intellectual functioning	Organic mental syndromes (acute brain syndrome- chronic brain syndrome) (measured by tests which reflect brain-cell loss [damage or dysfunction])
Situational experiential factors: family peers schooling occupation finances residence culture health and habits Personality factors: phenotype social ascriptions social achievements education occupation patterns of psychological emotional physical social adaptation	Interpersonal friction Disorders of thinking behavior affect	Reaction to loss of intellect Search for aid and support elaborated as: apathy pseudoanhedonia display of helplessness somatization hypochondriasis depression paranoid states explotive-manipulative states	Modification of life-long well-established mechanisms of psychological, emotional, social, and physical adjustment Behavior disorder or "neurosis" or, if genetic, diathesis and phenotypical propensity "Psychotic" disorder with signs of parasympathomimetic or sympathomimetic vegetative signs

*From Goldfarb, 1972.

Because of multiple sparing or aggravating effects on memory of previously established patterns of reaction, our clinical measures are rather reliable indicators predictive of mild, moderate and severe degrees of brain damage, but do not permit differentiations of degree within the area of moderate neuronal cell loss. Also, perceptual distortions (hallucinations) may at times accompany the defects of learning and memory in acute types; these are known as delirious states. The type and content of such deliriums, like the affect and thought disturbances that can complicate or be complicated by memory loss, are postdictively traceable to the previously acquired, well established mechanisms of adaptation and to genetic diatheses.

A decrease in functioning cells of the reticular formation appears, clinically, to be related to decrease in attention and to the awareness of being aware, to failure of central nervous system integrations contributing to that aspect of functioning called consciousness. This is seen as one type of acute organic brain syndrome: improved centroencephalic functioning results in reversal of the process -- recovery. When it is clinically present, the individual is vegetative. Thus, as cerebral cortex diminishes, there is memory loss; with decreasing memory, consciousness is lost; when the reticular formation (the centroencephalic grey matter) goes, the individual (as one aware of self and of living) dies, although he remains technically alive.

We live by memories; survival depends upon memory; memory is life. A sufficient decrease in memory can be expected to decrease likelihood of survival or, conversely, increase vulnerability to dying. Excellence of special care -- especially if institutionalized and including the use of so-called "institutions" -- better named protective settings, might counteract this but a sufficiently severe loss of memory can be expected to override even these efforts. That this is the case is shown after discussion of nosology and methods of measurement.

VI. CLASSIFICATION

In the foregoing remarks on clinical states, an old term, dementia, and the relatively new terms, acute organic brain syndrome and chronic organic brain syndrome, were introduced. The latter are categories or nosologic terms which are now current. Again, it must be emphasized, the conditions to which they refer should not be confused with disorders like the aphasias, agnosias and apraxias which can by some definition be considered to be loss of memory. These are organic mental states but are quite different from what are called organic brain syndromes as regards their etiology, course, implications for treatment and care, as well as in symptomatology. They may be, however, accompanied by organic brain syndrome when they are accompanied by diffuse cortical neuronal loss, and in end stages of organic brain syndrome aphasia, apraxia or agnosia may appear.

In the organic brain syndrome there is impaired mental functioning based upon a decreased capacity to learn and to remember. The irreversible form of this disorder, which we now call chronic, has long been referred to as dementia. The term denoted an acquired loss of mental capacity; it was a weakening of the memory, of the ability to learn and, perhaps, therefore, of reasoning. The German term for the disorder was "Schwachsinn", literally, weak or slight mind. Dementia occurring in old age came to be called senile dementia, somewhat redundantly perhaps in that the term senile already denotes infirmity and weakness of body or mind in contrast to the term senescence -- the state of being old. Categorization of senile psycho-organic changes, deterioration of mentation with increasing chronologic age, came to encompass more than weakness of remembering. The term came to connote the total derangement of the patient who might have concomitant affect, thought or overt behavioral disorders by attribution of these "personality" changes to the presumed structural damage or pathophysiology. In our psychiatric diagnostic groupings, the seemingly irreversible and progressive senile mental states, because of lack of clarity as to etiology, were first separated into the dementias of presumably toxic and metabolic deteriorative type and those of seemingly atherosclerotic cause. The first type was subdivided into subgroupings of "simple", presbyophrenic (again, old mind), delirious and confused (as it turns out, acute rather than chronic), depressed and agitated and paranoid. The cerebral arteriosclerosis type was included in psychiatric nosology as "with psychosis" and, once again, the types were to be specified as mood or thinking disorders. Such classification was scarcely truly indicative of etiology, and the careful outlining of onset, progression or course of the disorders and of the symptomatology was more based on belief, conviction and a Procrustean bed type of diagnostic skill than on the actual critical phenomena. There eventuated an agreement to call these conditions of seeming irreversible defects of remembering and learning chronic brain syndrome, while the reversible ones were to be called acute brain syndrome, each, so far as possible, to be listed according to presumed etiology. Following this, for semantic reasons, there was a decision to call these conditions organic brain syndromes, possibly because all mental syndromes must be referable to the brain as the organ of the mind. Again, in this clumsy attempt to point to the fact that these are conditions in which there is discernible structural brain damage, there was subdivision according to whether the presumed chief etiologic factors were metabolic, circulatory, genetic, endocrine dysfunction, intoxication, infection, drug or other; subdivision as to whether acute or chronic, and as to the type of mood or thought disorder present. What this amounts to, in sum, is that we recognize that there are many types of organically determined mental states; that one of these states which is subdivisible into acute and chronic forms is so common in old age as to be regarded as a disorder of old age; that this disorder is probably of multifactorial and multiple etiology. Many pathways may lead to the same common end in the case of the chronic form. This end is one of permanent memory loss and of decrement in ability to learn. Clinically this is characterized by memory loss, and inability to remain oriented for time, place or persons; these defects of learning and remembering are measurable by very simple tests of orientation and of general information, including the ability to do addition, subtraction and division. Whatever secondary signs may be present, such as deficiencies in reasoning, in judgment or with respect to affective display and lability, and whatever additional behavioral disturbance, such as alterations in sleep, eating and social participation may also be present, it is the defects in memory and learning that are basic to this condition. Inability to learn and poor memory are the common denominators of the differing manifestations related to changes in the brain common in chronological old age.

VII. MEASURES OF MEMORY LOSS

Tests of intellectual functioning, including memory and learning, are highly "contaminated" by the past experience of the individual. Such tests often do little more than tell us what an individual has had opportunities to learn, how he now learns and how well he remembers. They may not, however, make it possible for us to do more than estimate how much loss has occurred, and if we know little of the patient's past achievements, our estimate may be far off the mark. Usually the individual's vocabulary can help us assay his prior educational, occupational and intellectual achievement to which his present capacities for performance can be compared.

Tests of memory also may be invalidated because they do not differentiate between the poor performance of the

depressed, agitated, elated, hallucinatory or deluded person.
   In old age, even as in youth, alterations of motivation and physicochemical states related to mood changes may interfere with learning; such states may also result in spurious memory defects. Conversely, impairment of learning and memory may reduce apparent motivation and may superficially resemble changes in mood.
   Even mild emotional disturbances can influence cognitive functions. Tests of what one remembers, of how much one can remember that one now learns and for how long, will be as poorly done by a frightened, angry, depressed or uncooperative person as they would be if he had a slight to moderate degree of brain cell loss. Valid testing, therefore, must be done under conditions of good rapport with the patient in an optimal emotional and motivational state. The value and reliability of the test is, of course, enhanced if it is likely to yield valid information about the degree of brain inefficiency even when these conditions cannot be perfectly met. For this, a psychological measure, like a physical test, should be sensitive to brain damage, yield no false positives, be easily, quickly and comfortably performed and experienced, be easy to record and score, and require a minimum of fuss, apparatus, preparation or stage setting. Also, our tests should determine not only the presence but the severity of the disorder. In this respect, our evaluation should be concordant with the otherwise measurable, pathophysiologic, anatomical or neuropathologic features and the prognosis. Most simply put, our evaluation should point to etiology when possible, to prognosis and to treatment or care which can alter the course or decrease suffering (Goldfarb, 1969; Hurwitz, 1968).
   The foregoing illustrates the difficulties in devising a valid measure of memory loss with aging in old people. It has been possible, however, to validate two measures of gross memory loss. These are the specific groups of ten questions revealing the capacity to remain oriented for time and place and to remember recent and remote events. Also, a test of double-simultaneous stimulation appears to measure or reflect capacity to remember.
   With the help of Robert L. Kahn and Max Pollack, I learned that our clinical approach can be made more precise, more easily scored and better formulated for teaching purposes by the use of a ten-question procedure, which we began testing in 1958 (Kahn et al., 1960; Pollack et al., 1960; Pollack et al., 1962). Utilizing the data obtained by way of repeated yearly simultaneous physical, psychiatric and psychological examinations for ten years of about 1300 institutionalized

persons over 64 years of age, we validated what has come to be called the Mental Status Questionnaire (M.S.Q.). It was given this nickname because it was derived by determining which of about fifty questions in our mental status examination were most discriminatory with respect to the correct identification of persons with brain damage as confirmed by more complete examination and course of the disorder. This test and the areas presumptively tapped by it, is shown in Table III; the scoring I now prefer is shown in Table IV. At the same time, we found that double simultaneous stimulation of the face and hand -- nicknamed the "Face-Hand Test" (F.H.T.) (see Table V) -- was usually, but not always, concordant with the M.S.Q. When the F.H.T. was incorrectly done by persons who did relatively well with our "questionnaire", it occasionally revealed the presence of lesser memory defects, as confirmed by more extensive testing and the course of the disorder. The M.S.Q. may be misinforming as to the degree of brain damage present in persons -- like clerical workers -- who habitually remain well oriented for time and dates. Conversely, a poorly done M.S.Q. in a person who does the F.H.T. correctly may suggest the presence of poise, alertness and the presence of a capacity for optimal uses of resources, which may deceive the less careful examiner to believe there is less brain damage than is actually present. No one test tells us all. Information must be gathered in many ways and, from the medical point of view, artfully interpreted for practical purposes. The spelling of words with double consonants like "tract", "cart", "stack", "park", "crowd" or "seven", backwards as well as forwards, may reveal problems of short term, holding or rehearsal type of memory. Recitation of the alphabet, counting by twos or threes, and recitation of the months may reveal difficulties in concentration, tendencies to perseverate suggestive of other types of organic mental states. Surprisingly, the ability to hold and recite digits may be relatively good when diffuse cortical cell loss is present but poor when the person is depressed and attention and concentration are poor.

The seemingly simple test of memory called the M.S.Q. may have an extraordinary helpfulness in clinical practice. It can suggest that a patient will soon be in need of much care, that the outlook for life as well as for behavioral improvement is poor, and that the need for supervision and assistance is great. It can tell us the converse, in that the outlook for life may be good except as modified by underlying physical illness and that opportunities for behavioral improvement are considerable despite current need for supervision and assistance. Responses to the M.S.Q. may fluctuate within a narrow range, but there is no change in the score which can be attributed to learning unless the patient is improving. It is of interest that even though the patient may recall the questions he does not acquire the answers when brain damage is present. Marked fluctuation of the score is highly suggestive that the disorder has reversible aspects, that it is entirely "acute" or partially so. Thus, fluctuation of scores outside the "bands" in the M.S.Q. (3 to 5, 6 to 8, 9+) suggests a need for further investigation which may lead to definitive treatment. That is, the M.S.Q. score can be utilized as an index to improvement or worsening of the condition of persons with reversible memory loss.

Predictive Value of Measures of Memory Loss

I would like now to return to the matter of classification and to comment on the predictive value of memory loss with respect to course and longevity (see figures 2a and 2b). Survival in mentally ill old persons appears to be predictably related to psychiatric diagnosis as demonstrated by Kay, Norris, Post and Roth (Post, 1951; Hopkins and Roth, 1953; Kay and Roth, 1953; Kay et al., 1955; Roth, 1955; Kay et al., 1956; Kay, 1962). But, we found (Goldfarb, 1965) this was poorest if the diagnoses were made in terms of "Senile Dementia" and "Cerebral Arteriosclerosis with Psychosis". This appeared to be so because psychiatric judgment of the presence and degree of severity of each of these reactions is determined by observing the disturbed or disturbing nature of the person's reaction rather than to a basic impediment of cerebral function. The reaction type emerges from a conglomeration of personality factors, current situational strains or stresses, and the patient's hopes and expectations. Nevertheless, the presence of memory loss -- as attested to by the labeling of persons as demented, whatever the presumptive etiologic factors that led to the diagnosis of senility versus cerebral arteriosclerosis -- is predictive of a higher death rate as compared to persons free of such "organic" impairment whether or not mental disorder is present. But prediction of survival in persons labeled as demented is greatly sharpened by use of subclassifications which point to the degree of memory loss and to their probable permanent or temporary nature. If we use old popular terminology, persons called delirious and confused have a highest death rate (see Table VIII), and persons who fall into a group labeled Presbyophrenic Type or Simple Type of Senile Dementia have a higher death rate than persons classifiable as Depressed and Agitated or Paranoid with Dementia. Similarly, persons with so-called Cerebral Arteriosclerosis with little or no mood or affect disorder have a death rate lower than the group with Senile Dementias but higher than that for persons who have a "psychosis of affective or paranoid types" along with memory loss ascribed to cerebral vascular damage.

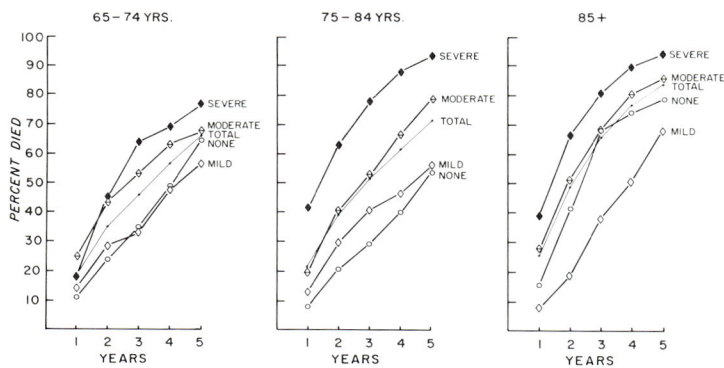

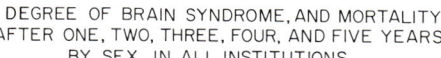

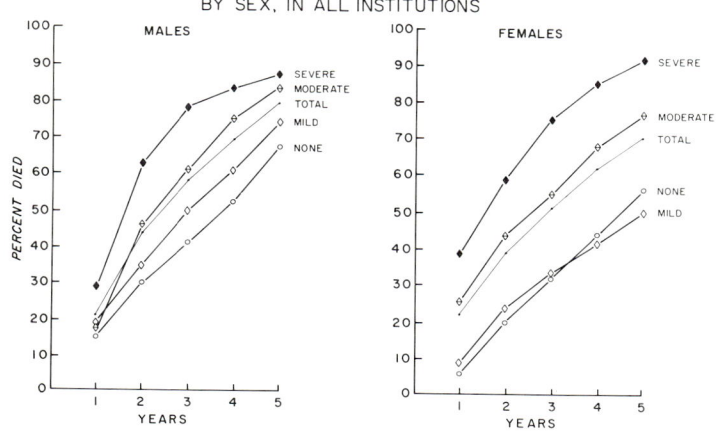

Fig. 2a

MSQ SCORE AND
MORTALITY AFTER ONE, TWO, THREE & FOUR YEARS

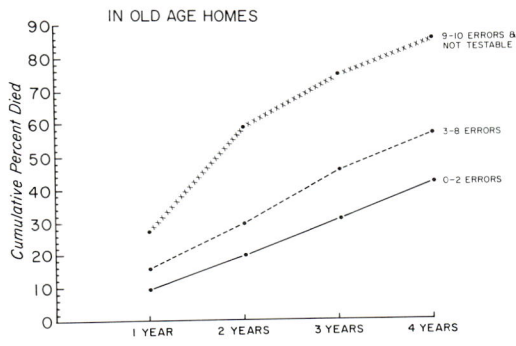

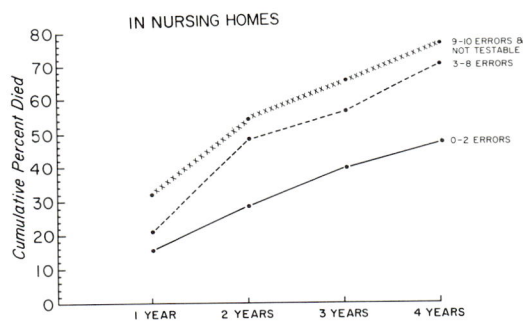

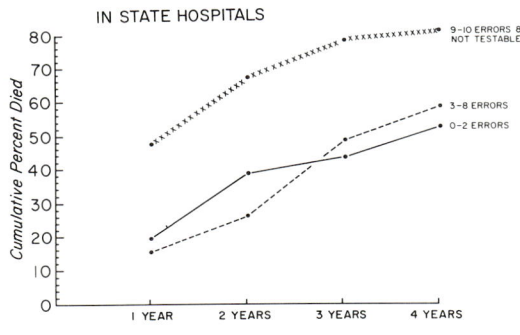

Fig. 2b

Table VIII

Death Rate in Percent for Each Year*

Category	Number	Year Examined						
		1	2	3	4	5	6	7
All persons	1,280	23	42	54	65	73	79	82
Male severe	426	23	44	58	69	78	83	87
Age 85+	290	28	52	68	79	90	92	92
Physical dependency, severe	257	37	63	74	82	88	93	95
Incontinent	244	38	61	75	84	92	95	97
MSQ Error 9+	424	35	60	73	83	89	93	94
Brain syndrome severe (psychiatrist diagnosis)	305	37	60	75	84	90	93	94

*From Goldfarb, 1969.

When the same patient's life expectancy is related to the measure of memory loss by M.S.Q., the predictive value is found to be more precise. Patients in whom there was coexistence of mood or thought disorder with memory loss had a better outlook for life than those in whom memory loss alone led to disorganization and disturbed or disturbing behavior. This tended to confirm our view that "it took brains" to elaborate a psychosis in old age and that psychiatrically depressed persons and paranoid persons had a lesser degree of memory and learning impairment. When we further classified these persons according to the severity of memory loss irrespective of associated disorder of mood, thought or behavior, the predictive value for life expectancy is greatly sharpened. Thus, our conviction that different populations with different life expectancy can be distinguished by tests of memory is confirmed.

What memory losses of the old are treatable and how can we treat them? If the memory loss is of the type determined by mood disorder, antidepressants are the cure. Even mild stimulants like Dextroamphetamine sulfate, properly buffered with a mild sedative, methyl phenidate in very small doses, or caffeine as the citrate or in coffee, can be helpful in motivating the patient, integrating efforts and decreasing apathy so that learning and memory improve. Where anger and fear act as "blocks" to good self utilization, there are many sedatives of value; among them is acetylsalicylic acid -- common aspirin -- barbiturates and the "tranquilizers" like the phenothiazines and thioridizine. When memory loss is of the type that reflects brain cell dysfunction and is reversible, treatment of the underlying condition is required. For the permanent memory loss that is related to brain cell loss with the concomitant diminution in the size and weight of the brain, we can do nothing more than favor optimal use of what is left; we can decrease the harmful effects of emergency emotion and help direct the person to optimal use of the remaining assets. Improvement of mood, motivation and alertness -- decrease of emergency emotion, and personal guidance toward the decrease of disorganized behavior or immobilization are goals which yield seeming -- although not necessarily measurable and real -- improvement in memory. An acute component is reduced in severity or, at least, remaining memory is made more accessible and is optimally used in reasoning and personal relations. As for the many treatments advanced by implication or clear statement, as ways of improving memory where the brain cells are gone, none of them appear to do this, although some of the drugs proposed may be mild antidepressants.

Implications for Treatment

It may be proper to conclude with an attempt to answer the question, what are the implications of what appear to be the facts about memory and aging?

There seems to be little or no hope for the restoration of learning ability and memory when this is a product of neuronal loss. There is no evidence that retraining or special forms of reorientation can result in the development of new circuitry or favor the improved use of old circuits when the damage has occurred. There are, at present, no vasodilators that have been shown to improve cerebral circulation. They may, in fact, make matters worse if circulation is the problem by way of stealing from the brain in need where the vessels are damaged by the brain not in need where the vessels can possibly react to the drug. Potassium iodide was, at one time, probably used in hopes that it improved circulation in atherosclerotic conditions; it was useless and is now largely forgotten. Glutamic acid did not prove of value. Based on the belief, from exciting experimental work with flatworms, that complex protein synthesis might provide answers, RNA substance by mouth and injection was used -- again, the results were not, despite early reports, encouraging. The histaminic substance serc does not help. Magnesium pemoline is of no established value for the reversal of such cognitive defect. Small amounts of amphetamines (1.25 mg, not 5 or 10 mg) and of methyl phenidate (1/2 mg, not 2 mg or 5 or 10 mg) may improve alertness and motivation as will caffeine in coffee or as caffeine citrate grs. 1/2 oz. once or twice a day. Metrazol has been advocated; its presumed action would be via increased respiratory efficiency leading to augmented oxygen pick-up by red blood cells and cause greatly improved cerebral support. Again, there has been no convincing support. "Hydergine", a mixture of adrenergic blocking dihydroergot oxines, has also been advanced for the improvement of the mental "senile" state, first on the basis of expecting to improve circulation, and later by way of more complex chemical actions on the nervous system: it appears to be ineffective insofar as improvement of memory is concerned. Recently, antioxidents -- Vitamin E -- have been advocated, but are of no value. Even more recently, because it appears to reduce lipofuscin in the cells, Lucidryl -- centrophenoxin -- has been thought of as possibly helpful: this remains to be demonstrated. "Gerovital" or "H_3", the brand names for Rumanian-manufactured Procaine HCl, has been advocated as a means to reverse the effects of senility. These claims have now been abandoned in this country, and it is now being advanced and tested for monoamine oxidase (MAO) inhibiting properties and as an antidepressant useful in "mild cases" of depression. So far, it is not of proven value. The use of hyperbaric oxygen could conceivably, at best, decrease reversible phenomena more easily done by other means. It may improve the oxygen carrying power of the blood where the oxygen carrying power has been decreased through bondage of red blood cells with carbon monoxide in smokers or persons exposed to highly polluted atmosphere. Such benefits could obviously be obtained by less expensive or potentially harmful personal or social changes. Also, high concentrations of oxygen can yield cerebral vascular constriction and, if prolonged, is toxic. L-Dopa, a catecholamine useful in Parkinsonism, appears to do nothing for the defects of memory and its coincidental defects of calculation and general information. This chemical may make disorders of mood worse and also add disturbance of thought. Further trial with this type of chemical is warranted, but so far it does not seem promising. Blood thinning compounds, considered to decrease "sludging", such as heparin, dicoumeral or aspirin, do not appear to be prophylactic and have not proven to be meliorative, despite such claims. Alcohol, as a protector against atherosclerosis by way of its capacity to decrease hepatic competence in destroying estrogens, would appear to be a heroic and misguided approach; in any case, the side effects might not be considered acceptable by many persons. RNA substances, by mouth or injection, have been of no proven value. What can be done in mild, moderate or moderately severe memory loss is the achievement of alteration of mood and improvement of overt behavior and, at times, of thought disorders where these are present. This can be done by decreasing fear and anger whether the emergency emotion be a reaction to the intellectual defect, to the changed social situation or the loss of role, status, money and ability. For this, personal relationships called psychotherapy (individual or group), antidepressant or anti-psychotic drugs and, at times, electro-shock therapy (E.S.T.) can be used. The value of protective settings -- usually congregate -- and prosthetic milieus cannot be overemphasized. At times, when the memory defect is severe, these must be provided despite the initial protest of the patient. When these facilities are good, they prove their worth by improving the patient, his outlook, and his appreciation of their value. Unfortunately, for the disorder of memory which is most clearly different from the senile states when it is noted to occur relatively early in life and was therefore called presenile dementia or Alzheimer's Disease, but which appears to be the process that lies behind most of the severe disorders of memory of the old -- about this we know nothing of prophylactic value.

What hope for the prophylaxis of memory defects is there now? The prevention of injury and infection, better systemic support of the old when ill or injured and during surgery may decrease the acceleration of senility in those doomed to develop it and may save many from unnecessary brain cell loss that may, if diffuse, result in a similar condition. Supervision of diet to provide adequate thiamine intake, and possibly nicotinic acid, avoidance of smoking, polluted air and insurance of adequate pulmonary ventilation may be ways of delaying what may be inevitable for some and avoiding the mild disorders entirely for others. Guarding against periods of low blood pressure, correction of anemia and reasonable control of diabetic states with avoidance of hypoglycemic episodes and prolonged periods of hyperglycemia or ketosis may make a difference. Avoidance of drug ingestion that leads to neuronal dysfunction, to hypoventilation or fall in blood pressure; the supervision of general health to guard against or correct cardiac failure, renal failure and azotemia whether primarily related to kidney disorder, hypertension and cardiovascular disease or diabetic nephrosis, and the quick correction of electrolyte disturbance related to these conditions, diuretics, dehydration, or other causes may be of help. In the search for remedial conditions, one must also remain aware that cerebral dysfunctions may be a symptom of cryptogenic neoplasms which are steroid producing like those of the adrenal cortex, in addition to more clear-cut disorders of the thyroid, parathyroid, and adrenal glands.

Although we apparently can do relatively little yet to prevent the occurrence of memory loss with illness and injury and probably nothing for that which appears to be genetically determined, it is nevertheless true that much can be done for melioration of mood, thinking and behavior of persons with memory losses. This is usually best provided in a good congregate protective care setting or prosthetic milieu. At times, this can be a one-bed psychiatric hospital and nursing home.

In all cases of disturbed orientation and decreased memory, an acute organic brain syndrome may complicate the chronic irreversible disorders. This complication can be avoided or reversed by attention to fluid balance, stabilization of pulmonary and cardiac function at optimal levels, care in the administration of drugs which directly or indirectly decrease cerebral competence, by regulation of sleep, bowel and bladder habits, insuring adequate diet, reasonable exercise, and the elimination of anxiety. There are also benefits to be derived from the rational use of cerebral, pulmonary and central nervous system stimulants in chronic organic brain syndrome to favor the optimal use of remaining physical and mental assets and to encourage their use by the alerting, motivating and euphorizing effects of the medications.

VIII. CONCLUDING REMARKS

In partial summary, memory decline is characteristic of the aging process. There appear to be several pathways to the memory loss through aging, among the most important are those which lead to the presenile and senile states known as dementia or Alzheimer's Disease. These may be joined by others that independently can lead to similar memory defects, but which alone would probably not progress to the same state of severity. This "non-Alzheimer" group includes the direct and indirect effects of infections, trauma, cardiovascular, pulmonary, hematologic and other diseases, impairments and accidents, "shock", as well as cerebrovascular accidents or cerebrovascular insufficiency of various types. Both the Alzheimer type - and there may be more than one, etiologically speaking - and the so-called toxic-metabolic-traumatic varieties may vary in emergence, evolution and course. They may begin as centrencephalic problems of decreased awareness which lead to decrease in registration, in learning and relearning, and in reinforcement of old information so that the individual is finally empty of memory; they may begin as defects of the areas in which registration normally occurs with the same end of memory loss and, finally, of awareness of self as well; they may begin with the loss of cortical integrative areas responsible for the holding and recreation of remembering; or cortex, mediencephalic and centrencephalic areas may be simultaneously involved. The puzzle and problem of how it is that old persons do not register or record information, of how it is that immediate memory suffers and there is decrease in learning ability and future memory stores, of how immediate and remote memory are related and how it is that remote memory is lost by decay, interference, non-availability or inaccessibility, stimulates the imagination and makes a fascinating investigative game of clinical work with the aged.

REFERENCES

Adams, G. F. (1974). In "Geriatric Medicine", pp. 135-145, Academic Press, New York.
Adams, R. D., Fischer, C. M., Hakim, S., Ojemann, R. G., and Sweet, W. H. (1965). New Eng. J. Med. 273, 117.
Allison, R. S. (1962). "The Senile Brain-A Clinical Study". Edward Arnold Publishers, Ltd., London.
Arenberg, D. (1967). The Gerontologist 7, 10.
Barr, D. P. (1955). In "Cerebral Vascular Diseases" (I. S. Wright, and E. H. Luckey, eds.), pp. 71, Grune and Stratton, New York.
Birren, J. E. (1964). "The Psychology of Aging". Prentice Hall, Inc., New Jersey.
Blessed, G., Tomlinson, B. E., and Roth, M. (1968). Brit. J. Psychiat. 114, 797.
Bogoch, S. (1968). "The Biochemistry of Memory". Oxford University Press, London.
Botwinick, J. (1967). "Cognitive Processes in Maturity and Old Age". Springer Publishing Co., New York.
Bourne, G. H. (1973). In "Neurobiological Aspects of Maturation and Aging" (D. H. Ford, ed.), Prog. Brain Res. 40, 187, Elsevier Scientific Publishing Co., Amsterdam.
Brody, H. (1973). In "Development and Aging in the Nervous System" (M. Rockstein, and M. L. Sussman, eds.), pp. 121-133, Academic Press, New York.
Cherkin, A. (1965). Proc. Nat. Acad. Sci. 55, 88.
Cherkin, A. (1969). Proc. Nat. Acad. Sci. 63, 1094.
Corsellis, J. A. N. (1962). "Mental Illness and the Aging Brain". Oxford University Press, London.
De Jong, R. N., Itabashi, H. H., and Olson, J. R. (1969). Arch. Neurol. 20, 339.

Ehrentheil, O. F. (1957). *Geriatrics* 12, 428.
Essman, W. B., and Nakajima, S. (eds.) (1973). "Current Biochemical Approaches to Learning and Memory". Spectrum Publications, New York.
Fields, W. S. (1972). In "Aging and the Brain" (C. M. Gaitz, ed.), pp. 135-143, Plenum Press, New York.
Fisher, C. M., and Adams, R. D. (1964). *Acta Neurol.Scandinav.* 40, 9.
Foley, J. M. (1972). In "Aging and the Brain" (C. M. Gaitz, ed.), pp. 153-161, Plenum Press, New York.
Gellerstedt, N. (1933). "Zur Kenntnis der Hirnveranderungen bei der Normalen Altersinvolution". Uppsala: Almquist and Wiksells Boktryckeri-A-B.
Geschichter, C. F. (1959). VA Research in Aging Prospectus, U.S. Veterans Administration, Washington, D. C.
Goldfarb, A. I. (1957). *J. Chronic Diseases* 6, 483.
Goldfarb, A. I. (1964a). Unpublished.
Goldfarb, A. I. (1964b). In "Evaluation of Psychiatric Treatment" (P. H. Hoch, and J. Zubin, eds.), pp. 271-280, Grune and Stratton, New York.
Goldfarb, A. I. (1965). *J. Occupational Med.* 7, 499.
Goldfarb, A. I. (1969). *Arch. Gen. Psychiat.* 21, 172.
Goldfarb, A. I. (1971). In "Prediction of Lifespan" (E. Palmore, and F. C. Jeffers, eds.), pp. 79-93, D. C. Heath and Co., Lexington, Massachusetts.
Goldfarb, A. I. (1972). In "Aging and the Brain" (C. M. Gaitz, ed.), pp. 180, Plenum Press, New York.
Goldfarb, A. I. (1973). *Bull. N.Y. Acad. Med.* 49, 1070.
Goldfarb, A. I., and Antin, S. (1974). Unpublished data.
Goldfarb, A. I., and Fisch, M. (1964). *The Gerontologist* 4, 21.
Goldfarb, A. I., and Jahn, J. A. (1959). Unpublished report.
Goldfarb, A. I., Fisch, M., and Gerber, I. E. (1966). *Diseases Nervous System* 27, 21.
Grunthal, E. (1931). *Ztschr. Neurol. Psychiat.* 136, 464.
Guze, S., and Cantwell, D. (1964). *Am. J. Psychiat.* 120, 9.
Hopkins, B., and Roth, M. (1953). *J. Mental Sci.* 99, 451.
Hurwitz, L. J. (1968). *Gerontol. Clin.* 10, 146.
Inglis, J. (1957). *J. Mental Sci.* 103, 796.
Jahn, J. A. (1975). Personal communication.
Jarvick, L. F., and Cohen, D. (1973). In "The Psychology of Adult Development and Aging" (C. E. Eisdorfer, and M. P. London, eds.), American Psychological Association, Washington, D. C.
John, E. R. (1967). "Mechanisms of Memory". Academic Press, New York.
Kahn, R. L., Goldfarb, A. I., Pollack, M., and Peck, A. (1960). *Am. J. Psychiat.* 117, 326.

Kay, D. (1962). *Acta Neurol. Scandinav.* 38, 249.
Kay, D., and Roth, M. (1955). *Lancet* 269, 740.
Kay, D., Roth, M., and Hopkins, B. (1955). *J. Mental Sci.* 101, 302.
Kay, D., Norris, V., and Post. F. (1956). *J. Mental Sci.* 102, 129.
Kety, S. S. (1960). *Science* 132, 1861.
Kiev, A., Chapman, L. F., Guthrie, T. C., and Wolff, H. G. (1962). *Neurology* 12, 385.
Kral, V. A. (1962). *Can. Med. Assoc. J.* 86, 257.
Kral, V. A. (1972). *Can. Med. Assoc. J.* 108, 584.
Lassen, N. E. (1961). *Neurology* 11, 41.
Lauter, H., and Meyer, J. E. (1968). *In* "Senile Dementia" (C. Muller, ed.), pp. 13-26, Hans Huber Publishers, Bern and Stuttgart.
Malamud, N. (1972). *In* "Aging and the Brain" (C. M. Gaitz, ed.), pp. 63-87, Plenum Press, New York.
Obrist, W. D. (1972). *In* "Aging and the Brain" (C. M. Gaitz, ed.), pp. 117-133, Plenum Press, New York.
Worm-Petersen, J., and Pakkenberg, H. (1968). *J. Gerontol.* 23, 445.
Pollack, M., Kahn, R. L., Gerber, I., and Goldfarb, A. I. (1960). *Am. J. Psychiat.* 117, 120.
Pollack, M., Goldfarb, A. I., and Kahn, R. L. (1962). *In* "Social and Psychological Aspects of Aging" (C. W. Tibbitts, and W. Donahue, eds.), pp. 606-614, Columbia University Press, New York.
Post. F. (1951). *Brit. Med. J.* 1, 436.
Razran, G. (1971). "Mind in Evolution". Houghton Mifflin Co., Boston.
Roth, M. (1955). *J. Mental Sci.* 101, 281.
Roth, M. (1971). *In* "Recent Developments in Psychogeriatrics" (D. W. K. Kay, and A. Walk, eds.), Headley Bros., Ashford, England.
Roth, M., Tomlinson, B. E., and Blessed, G. (1966). *Nature* 209, 109.
Rothschild, D. (1937). *Am. J. Psychiat.* 93, 757.
Rothschild, D. (1942). *Arch. Neurol. Psychiat.* 48, 417.
Simon, A., and Malamud, N. (1965). "Psychiatric Disorders in the Aged". Geigy, Ltd., Manchester, England.
Sjögren, T., Sjögren, H., and Lindgren, A. G. H. (1952). *Acta. Psychiat. Neurol. Scand.*, Suppl. No. 82, pp. 1-125.
Smythis, J. R., Coppen, A., and Kreitman, N. (1968). "Biological Psychiatry". William Heineman Medical Books, London.
Strauss, H., Ostow, M., and Greenstein, L. (1952). "Diagnostic Electroencephalography". Grune and Stratton, New York.

Talland, G. A., and Wauch, N. C. (eds.) (1969). "The Pathology of Memory". Academic Press, New York.

Terry, R. D., and Wisniewski, H. M. (1972). In "Aging and the Brain" (C. M. Gaitz, ed.), pp. 89-116, Plenum Press, New York.

Victor, M., Adams, R. D., and Collins, G. H. (1971). "The Wernicke-Korsakoff Syndrome", Contemporary Neurology Series, pp. 138-139, F. A. Davis Co., Philadelphia.

Weil, A. (1945). "Textbook of Neuropathology". Grune and Stratton, New York.

Wells, C. E. (ed.) (1971). "Dementia", Contemporary Neurology Series, F. A. Davis Co., Philadelphia.

Whittier, J. R. (1974). Presented at the Annual Review Research Symposium on Psychopharmacology at the Psychiatric Institute, May 14, 1974.

Whittier, J. R., and William, D. (1956). J. Nervous Mental Disease 124, 618.

Willanger, R., Thygesen, P., Nielsen, R., and Petersen, O. (1968). Danish Med. Bull. 15, 65.

Wolstenholme, G. E. W., and O'Connor, M. (1970). "Alzheimer's Disease and Related Conditions". J. A. Churchill, London.

AGING AND SLEEP

Joyce D. Kales, M.D.*

Associate Director, Sleep Research and
Treatment Center and
Assistant Professor, Department of Psychiatry
Pennsylvania State University
Milton S. Hershey Medical Center
Hershey, Pennsylvania 17033

Prior to the advent of the modern era of sleep research, studies in aging focused primarily on the waking individual. In the early 1950's Aserinsky and Kleitman (1953) and Dement and Kleitman (1957) discovered that sleep consisted of a series of qualitatively different events recurring periodically throughout the night. These discoveries and subsequent studies that contributed to our basic understanding of sleep and dream patterns have provided investigators with another valuable tool for studying the physical and intellectual changes seen in aging.

In general, physicians focus most of their attention on a patient's daytime symptomatology and often pay little attention to the patient's complaints of disturbed sleep. Perhaps much of this is accounted for by the fact that sleep has long been regarded as a fairly uniform, quiescent, stress-free state. However, this is not the case. Each night of sleep is characterized by several distinct cyclical patterns which are well defined and can be demonstrated with great precision in the sleep laboratory by electrophysiologic techniques.

TECHNIQUES OF SLEEP RESEARCH

A fairly uniform methodology is utilized by the more than two dozen sleep laboratories in the United States. In these laboratories, precise profiles of sleep are determined for normal subjects and patients with various disorders. Data

---

*Jointly with Anthony Kales, M.D., Director, Sleep Research and Treatment Center, and Professor and Chairman, Department of Psychiatry, Pennsylvania State University, Milton S. Hershey Medical Center.

collection is primarily based on electroencephalographic (EEG), electroöculographic (EOG) and electromyographic (EMG) tracings from subjects or patients who are studied nightly for 7 to 10 hour periods. Standard electrode placements are made on the scalp to detect brain activity, at the outer canthus of each eye to record eye movements, and beneath the chin to determine muscle tonus. Other electrodes also monitor heart and respiratory rate. These electrical potentials are then transmitted to the polygraphic recorders. Later, the complete sleep recordings for each night are individually analyzed (Rechtschaffen and Kales, 1968).

Several consecutive laboratory nights of recording are required to obtain a complete profile of the sleep patterns characteristic of the particular entity being studied. There is a well established adaptation effect to the sleep laboratory consisting of a decrease in rapid eye movement (REM) in sleep and an increase in total wakefulness (Agnew et al., 1966). As a consequence, subjects are allowed to sleep for one or two nights in the laboratory to adapt to sleeping in this new environment. Baseline measurements for the particular study are established on the third and fourth nights. By comparing these baseline nights to those of normal subjects in the same age group, investigators can determine the effects of various conditions on sleep as well as the effect of sleep on these conditions. In some studies, the subjects or patients are monitored for a number of nights beyond the baseline nights in order to assess effects of various experimental manipulations or therapeutic procedures such as drug administration that may cause changes in the subject's sleep.

SLEEP PATTERNS

Sleep Stages

Normal sleep is divided into two main categories comprising a total of five stages (Rechtschaffen and Kales, 1968). Nonrapid eye movement (or NREM) sleep includes stages 1, 2, 3 and 4. Rapid eye movement (or REM) sleep is the fifth stage and is also called stage REM, active sleep or paradoxical sleep (figure 1).

In the awake stage, the electroencephalographic tracings show a low amplitude, mixed frequency activity, electroöculographic activity is present and electromyographic activity is at its highest levels.

NREM Sleep - In stage 1 sleep there is an absence of rapid eye movements and the EEG pattern is of low amplitude, irregular fast frequency activity.

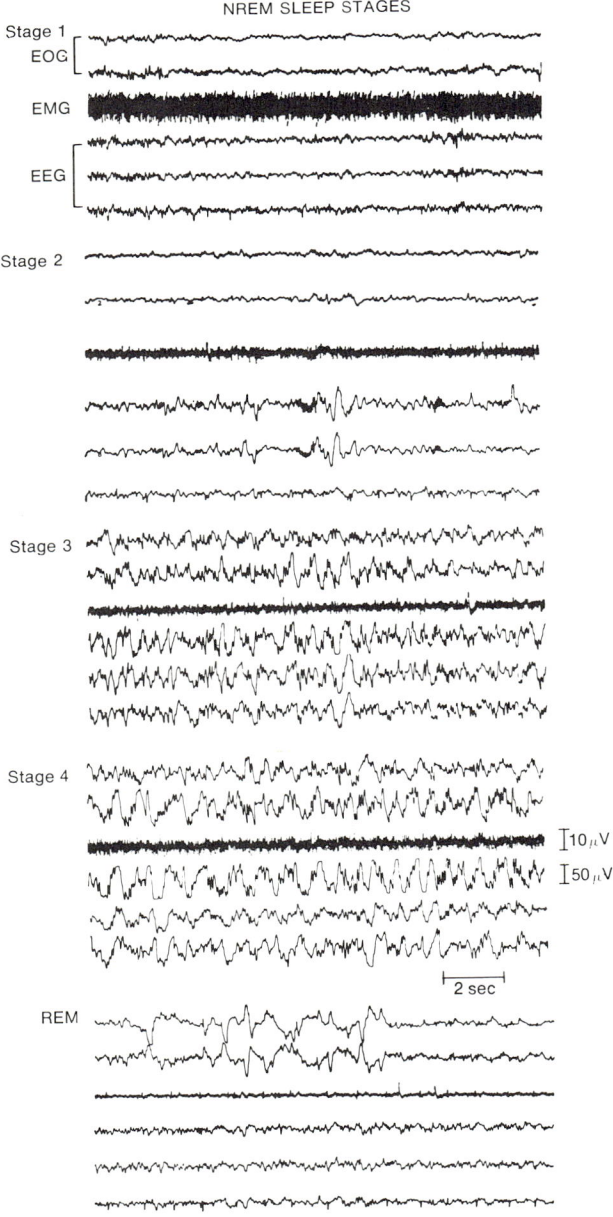

Fig. 1 Sleep Stages. The same six channels are used throughout, as labeled in the stage 1 record. Electroöculogram (EOG): eye movements: . . . . . (continued on page 190)

Fig. 1 (continued) . . . . electromyogram (EMG): muscle tonus from beneath the chin. Note the high EMG and eye movements in the awake state, the absence of rapid eye movements (REM's) in stage 1 (NREM), and REM's with decreased muscle tonus during REM sleep; stages 2, 3 and 4 show progressive slowing of frequency and increase in amplitude of the electroencephalogram. (From Kales, 1968.)

In stage 2 sleep, there are wave forms known as spindles of 12 to 16 cycles/second which occur against a background of low amplitude, fast frequency activity.

In stage 3 sleep, there are high amplitude, slow frequency waves that comprise 20 to 50 percent of the EEG record. When these slow waves make up 50 percent or more of the EEG record, stage 4 sleep is reached.

In NREM sleep, eye movements are absent and muscle tonus is reduced only slightly to moderately from the waking state.

REM Sleep - REM sleep is characterized by low amplitude, fast frequency EEG activity. Bursts of eye movements are present. Just prior to or at the onset of a REM period, muscle tonus shows a sudden, marked decrease which is sustained throughout the REM period except for brief, phasic activity.

Sleep Cycle for a Normal Young Adult - A typical night of sleep (figure 2) begins with stage 1 and is followed by stages 2, 3 and 4, respectively. Then, there is a return from stage 4 to stages 3 and 2. About 70 to 100 minutes after sleep onset, the individual enters the first period of REM sleep. After this REM period which is brief in duration, the individual completes another cycle descending through stages 2, 3 and 4 and ascending through stages 3, 4 and again returning to REM sleep. This cycling from the onset of one period of REM sleep through to the onset of the next period of REM sleep is repeated through the night. The pattern of sleep is similar throughout the night with the exception that during the latter part of the night, REM periods lengthen and the descent of sleep only reaches stage 2 or stage 3, from which there is the return to REM sleep (Dement and Kleitman, 1957).

Each night, the number of cycles and REM periods varies between 4 and 6 depending on the length of sleep. Twenty to 25 percent of total sleep time is spent in REM sleep; 50 percent in stage 2; 20 percent in stages 3 and 4; and 5 to 10 percent in stage 1.

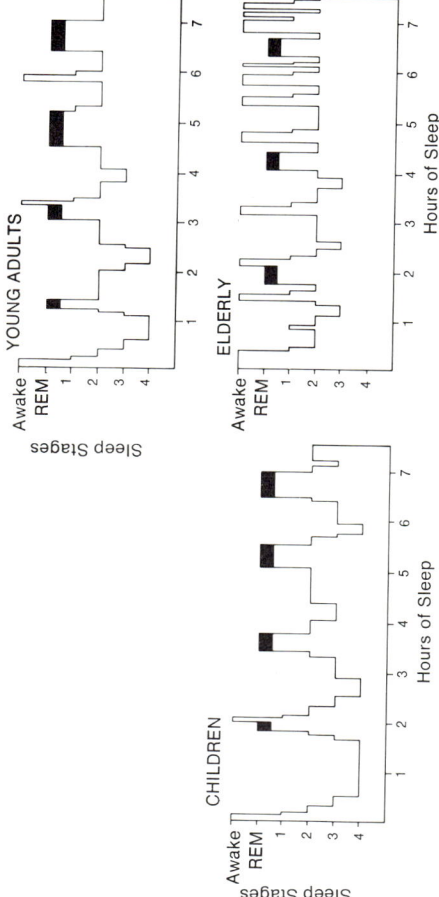

Fig. 2 Sleep Cycles and Age. The sleep of children and young adults shows early preponderance of stages 3 and 4, progressive lengthening of the first three REM periods, and infrequent awakenings. In elderly adults, there is little or no stage 4 sleep, REM periods are fairly uniform in length, and awakenings are frequent and often lengthy. (From Kales, 1968.)

JOYCE D. KALES

EFFECTS OF AGE ON SLEEP

The aging process affects sleep in three major areas; length, distribution in a 24 hour day and sleep stage patterns (Webb, 1970). Average sleep length decreases from 16 hours at birth to 12 hours plus a one hour nap at 2-3 years, 10 hours at 8-12 years, 8 hours in young adults and significantly less in the elderly due to frequent and prolonged awakenings.

In terms of sleep distribution, the sleep of the neonate is polyphasic. By the first year, naps tend to consolidate into a single afternoon nap and then do not regularly reoccur until advanced age, often making an assessment of total sleep time difficult.

Sleep stage patterns also undergo considerable change throughout the aging process (Roffwarg et al., 1964). There is no differentiation of NREM sleep into stages until after the first year of life. Premature and newborn infants show the highest percentage of REM sleep (Parmalee et al., 1967); the range is from 85 percent at 29 weeks conceptional age to 40 percent at 53 weeks. During the first year of life, REM sleep decreases to 20 to 25 percent of total sleep.

While the percentage of REM sleep remains in the range of 20 to 25 percent throughout life, stages 3 and 4 sleep (slow wave sleep) decrease progressively.

In children, the combined percentage of stages 3 and 4 sleep is high, comprising about 20 to 30 percent of total sleep time. In young adults, the percentage of slow wave sleep decreases to 10 to 20 percent.

In older subjects, the middle-aged and elderly, there is a further decrease in slow wave sleep with stage 4 sleep being virtually absent in the elderly (Feinberg et al., 1967; Kales et al., 1967). In addition, there is a substantial decrease in total sleep time because of frequent and often lengthy awakenings. Thus, in the elderly, sleep is both quantitatively and qualitatively different from that which they experienced earlier in their lives.

While the percentage of REM sleep in the normal elderly is similar to other age groups, there are certain alterations in REM sleep parameters, perhaps related to the marked decrease in stage 4 sleep. The time from sleep onset to the first REM period (REM latency) is shortened and the length of the first REM period is increased compared to the normal young adult. In the normal young adult, the greater amount of stage 4 sleep and the possible need for stage 4 sleep may account for the longer latency to the first REM period as well as its shorter length (Feinberg, 1969).

Sleep alterations in the elderly are not only indicated

by an increase in wakefulness and decrease in slow wave sleep, but also by frequent interruptions of REM sleep and the occurrence of poorly formed spindles in NREM sleep (Kahn and Fisher, 1969a). The REM sleep interruptions are due to intrusions of stage 2 sleep into the REM sleep period. In NREM sleep, the spindles are not only poorly formed but appear less frequently and their frequencies are often below the 12 to 14 cps range seen in normal young adults. This frequency reduction is similar to the reduction in the alpha rhythm frequency seen with aging.

Chronic Brain Syndrome

In comparing young and aged normal subjects and patients with chronic brain syndrome (CBS), Feinberg et al. (1967) noted that normal aging is associated with decreased total sleep, decreased stage 4, and a tendency toward a decrease in REM sleep. Pathological aging, as manifested by the CBS group, resulted in an accentuation of these changes. Within the CBS group, total sleep time was highly and significantly correlated with scores of intellectual function, i.e., with lowered intellectual functioning there was less total sleep time. In addition to these findings, several CBS subjects awakened regularly from REM sleep in states of agitation and delirium lasting 5 to 10 minutes and had to be physically restrained. It was suggested that the regularly occurring delirious behavior of these CBS patients, arising from awakenings from REM sleep, may represent a relationship between REM sleep and the syndrome of nocturnal delirium and wandering. This syndrome may reflect the inability of an impaired cerebrum to distinguish between dreaming and reality.

DREAMING

The traditional concept of dreaming has been that it is a randomly occurring and unpredictable experience. Aserinsky and Kleitman (1953) questioned whether this unique sleep stage was the one in which dreaming occurred. When they awakened subjects from REM sleep periods, vivid dreams were recalled 74 percent of the time but only 7 percent of the time from NREM awakenings. The high incidence of dream recall following REM sleep awakenings has been confirmed in many studies. This finding has led to REM sleep also being referred to as "dreaming sleep". In NREM sleep, the mental activity that occurs appears more closely related to thinking rather than dreaming and is more likely to be a manifestation of one's daily preoccupations.

A number of factors affect the frequency and detail of dream recall. Dream recall decreases in proportion to the amount of time elapsing from the end of a REM period to the awakening. Investigators found that when more than eight minutes elapsed from the end of the REM period to the awakening, dream recall was essentially absent (Dement and Wolpert, 1958). This suggests that brief, spontaneous awakenings during REM sleep may be necessary for memory consolidation and are one factor affecting an individual's ability to recall dreaming upon awakening in the morning.

The depth of sleep and length of REM periods also affect dream recall. The depth of sleep as determined by the auditory awakening threshold is higher early in the sleep period when stages 3 and 4 predominate and much lower later in the night when stage 2 and REM sleep predominate (Rechtschaffen et al., 1966). In addition, the first REM period is brief in duration, i.e., 5-10 minutes compared to subsequent REM periods later in the night which average 20 to 30 minutes. Thus, dreams from REM periods occurring later in the sleep period are more easily recalled and are more detailed, whereas dreams from the first REM period are poorly recalled and are fragmented in detail (Rechtschaffen et al., 1963).

Among any group of individuals, there are those who indicate that they recall dreams frequently and others who not only do not recall any specific dreams but insist that they never dream. Two groups of subjects, one with a history of recall in dreams frequently, and another recalling dreams rarely, were evaluated to see if there were any differences in their dream recall following awakenings in the sleep laboratory (Goodenough et al., 1959). REM periods occurred with equal frequency in both groups. Although the frequency of recall from awakenings made during REM periods was greater for the recallers, the non-recallers still reported dreams from about half of the REM awakenings.

Dream Recall in the Elderly

Weisz (1969) conducted a pilot study to determine the frequency and content of dreams reported following awakenings from REM sleep in the aged. Four elderly male subjects had their sleep monitored in the sleep laboratory for four nonconsecutive nights in the laboratory. Dream reports were rated by the author on six dimensions (Vivid Fantasy, Active Control, Hedonic Tone, Verbal and Physical Aggression and Sex).

There were a total of 55 awakenings; 64 percent of the REM sleep awakenings produced some substantive recall, while only 13 percent of the NREM awakenings resulted in dream recall. There was considerable inter-subject variability in dream recall from REM sleep awakenings, with a range from 20 to 100 percent. Dream reports contained more recreational and social themes than any other single category. There were only a few dreams with clear cut temporal regression, and these usually took the form of a friend, rather than the subject himself. The most striking feature of the dream content was the relatively passive participation of the dreamer. The dreamer tended to be the receiver of others' actions or an observer of events around him rather than an initiator of action. A diminished level of impulse expression was suggested by the generally low ratings for sexuality and verbal and physical aggression.

In another sleep laboratory dream recall study (Kahn and Fisher, 1967), fifty-eight REM period awakenings were made in 11 healthy aged male subjects, ages 70 to 87 years, over a total of 18 subject nights. Of these REM awakenings, 38 percent resulted in dream recall. The 38 percent recall was significantly lower ($p < .001$) than the 87 percent recall reported by the same investigators for young adults. The dream content from these REM sleep awakenings was not manifestly concerned with lost resources or increased frustrations as have been previously reported by Altshuler et al. (1963), who evaluated daytime dream recall reports in the elderly.

In their study, Altshuler and his associates conducted a comprehensive evaluation of dream content in the elderly. Volunteers over age 65 were obtained in a New York City day center for the aged. Many of the dreams reported seemed to have direct reference to concern about lost resources for coping with problems. There was no other clearly defined single category; the remainder of the dreams were categorized as miscellaneous but generally were concerned with the active pursuit of goals.

Several of the day center elderly subjects in this study presented dreams very similar to those of institutionalized aged subjects previously studied by the same investigators (Barad et al., 1961). The major theme was that of lost resources with or without a clear indication of a wish for restoration of powers. The content of these dreams included the following themes; wandering in a strange place, being lost or unable to find a way, looking for help, being left behind, or losing something familiar. The affect in these dreams was recalled as an uncomfortable vague sense of apprehension, confusion, uncertainty, or strangeness.

In the dreams classified as miscellaneous, the dreamer saw himself as being active in the pursuit of a goal in contrast to the oral themes of wishful passivity coupled with helplessness so frequently represented in the dreams of lost resources.

As mentioned, the same investigators conducted another study (Barad et al., 1961) of dream content with subjects in a home for the aged where 80 percent had chronic brain syndrome of some degree. Their findings suggested that dreams of lost resources are associated with the existence or development of organic brain changes. In comparing the findings from these institutionalized patients and from the non-institutionalized day center subjects, the authors suggest that dreams of this type in aged persons may be qualified evidence of chronic brain syndrome or its incipient development.

SEXUALITY IN THE AGING

The association between penile erections and REM sleep illustrates the relationship between psychological and physiological processes of dreaming.

Penile erections are often temporally related to REM sleep (Fisher et al., 1965). In normal subjects, penile erections invariably begin and end in close temporal proximity to the onset and termination of REM periods. Actually, penile erections begin several minutes before the onset of REM sleep, suggesting that a neurophysiological mechanism initiates the penile erection prior to the development of any dream content. The "morning" or "bladder" erection probably was previously thought to be primarily related to urinary pressure or sexual dream content. We now know that its presence or absence depends most upon whether one awakens from REM or NREM sleep. While all of these points emphasize the physiological correlates of REM sleep, the regular occurrence of penile erections during this phase of sleep may in itself act as a stimulus for initiating sexual content into the ongoing dream material, i.e., the physiology affecting the psychology.

Kahn and Fisher (1969b) studied eighteen healthy male subjects, ages 71 to 96 years, for three or two nights each while measuring penile erection with a mercury strain gauge. For this group, 45 percent of the REM periods were categorized as having full or moderate erection and the remaining 55 percent had slight or no erections. The 45 percent REM erection frequency for the aged is less than the 83 percent reported by Fisher et al. (1965) and the 80 percent reported by Karacan et al. (1966) both in the young adult. There was considerable variance in this group of elderly subjects and a number did not demonstrate reduced erection. Five of the twelve subjects, ages 71 to 80, had REM sleep erections similar to those reported for young adults. Thus, the investigators noted that although amount of REM erection is lowered in the 70's, in individual cases it may be maintained as late as 80 to a degree approximating that of the young man. Of the three oldest subjects, ages 87, 95 and 96, two still exhibited some REM erection, but this was reduced to about one-third of full circumference change.

INSOMNIA IN THE ELDERLY

The symptom of insomnia is frequently present in any condition where pain, discomfort, fear, anxiety or depression are prominent factors. In many conditions, several of these factors co-exist and insomnia is even more likely to be present. The five conditions which account for the vast majority of difficulties with insomnia are Situational Stresses or Crises, Medical Conditions, Psychological Disorders, Drug Withdrawal Insomnia and the Aging Process (Kales et al., 1974a).

In the aging process, many of the factors mentioned before may contribute to the sleep difficulty. Medical illnesses with pain and discomfort are of course much more frequent in the elderly. In addition, the realities of declining function and inevitable death, create to varying degrees in the elderly fear, anxiety and depression.

Insomnia may consist of difficulty in falling asleep, difficulty in staying asleep, early final awakening or any combination of these (figure 3). We were interested in determining the incidence of insomnia in the general population as well as determining how the incidence changes with age. To answer both these questions, we devised a number of statements relating to sleep difficulty for inclusion in the Los Angeles Metropolitan Area Survey (LAMAS) (Kales et al., 1974a). We found that the incidence of a current complaint of sleep difficulty within this representative sample was 32 percent. Moreover, the incidence of a complaint of insomnia at any time during the repondent's life was 41.9 percent.

The age distribution of the respondents reporting insomnia was significantly different from that of the total sample. In the youngest age range (18-29), the respondent complained less frequently of insomnia, while the complaint of insomnia was more frequent in the older respondent (above 60 years). When both sex and age were considered, additional differences were noted. Insomnia was less frequent in young males and more frequent in older females than would have been expected from the total sample distribution.

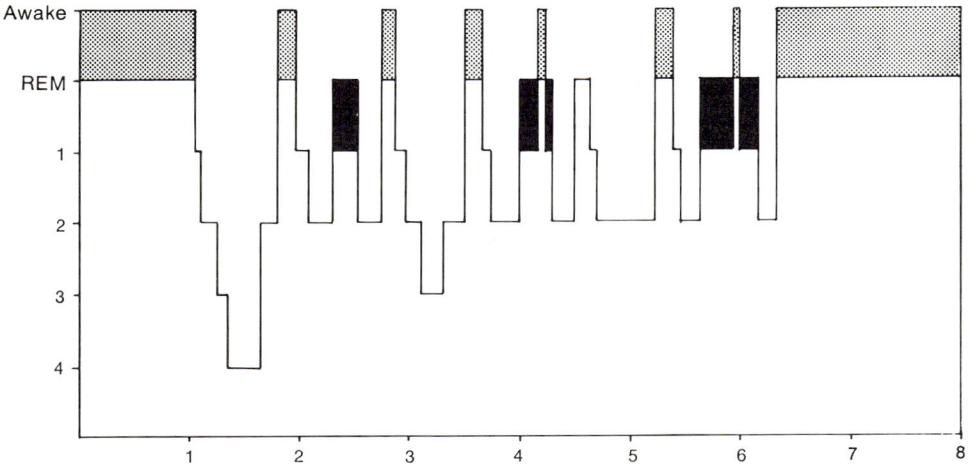

Fig. 3 Sleep patterns in insomnia. Depicted are a composite of three different types of insomnia: difficulty falling asleep, difficulty staying asleep, difficulty staying asleep (with frequent awakenings), and early final awakening. Insomnia may consist of one, or a combination, of these difficulties. (From Kales et al., 1974b.)

Analysis of the first 124 insomniac patients seen in our Sleep Disorders Clinic showed a high degree of psychopathology in the group. Minnesota Multiphasic Personality Inventories (MMPI's) demonstrated that 85 percent of the patients had one or more scales elevated to the pathological range. The most frequently elevated scales were depression, conversion hysteria, psychasthenia and schizophrenic trends (Kales and Kales, 1972).

The most outstanding feature of this insomniac sample in terms of psychopathology was the high occurrence of depression. In addition to Scale 2 (or the depression scale) being the single most frequently elevated scale, it was also among the three highest scales in 96 percent of all of the patients with elevated profiles.

There were marked differences in the depression patterns for these insomniac patients when different age groups of the patients were compared. In the age group of under 30 years, 54 percent had depression patterns. One pattern type accounted for many of the depression profiles and was characterized by an intellectualized, schizoid depression with an identity-disturbed profile. In the 30-49 year age group, 71 percent had depression patterns with three particular depression patterns being predominant. One pattern was the same as that described for the under 30 years group. The other two pattern types are associated with anxiety and depression in passive-dependent personalities and somatized depression where health is a major preoccupation. In the 50 and older group, 82 percent had depression patterns. There was one major pattern in this group, the somatic depression pattern which is characterized by apprehensions and anxieties about health.

Thus, the depression in the younger insomniacs appears to be qualitatively different from that in older insomniacs. These MMPI patterns also suggest that the younger patients more readily admit their depressions, anxieties, and self-doubts and are more willing to see their insomnia as related to their being depressed. The older patients are much more likely to focus on their sleep symptoms so as to avoid facing their underlying if not more overt depressions (Kales and Kales, 1972). The treatment of insomnia in the elderly patient depends upon a number of factors including the type of psychological disturbance underlying the symptom and whether medical conditions such as coronary artery disease are also present. The treatment may be directed toward alleviating the symptom, the underlying psychological disturbance or both.

In those neurotic, anxious patients in whom depression is not a significant factor, the treatment is symptomatic, utilizing hypnotic drugs. Where the problem of insomnia is either transient or mild and only short term drug therapy is indicated, virtually any hypnotic drug can be used. Most hypnotics are quite effective in inducing and maintaining sleep for short periods of time, *i.e.*, for approximately one week of therapy. In most insomniac patients, where intermediate and long term drug therapy is indicated, flurazepam (Dalmane) is the drug of choice. Sleep laboratory studies have demonstrated that in contrast to other hypnotic drugs, which become ineffective after one or two weeks of administration, flurazepam continues to be effective. In the elderly, treatment is frequently initiated with 15 mg at bedtime. After 7 to 10 days of therapy, if the insomnia is not alleviated, the dosage may be increased to 30 mg, if tolerated (Kales and Kales, 1974a).

In those elderly patients where depression is a significant aspect underlying the insomnia, antidepressant medication is used. Because of the negative inotropic effects and production of occasional tachycardia produced by the tricyclic antidepressant drugs, caution is indicated when treating patients with coronary artery disease. Usually an antidepressant drug with a sedative side effect is most effective in treating the depression and symptom of insomnia when given in a large dose at bedtime. A large dose at bedtime should not be used initially, but rather, the physician should prescribe a small dose such as 25 mg of the drug and gradually increase the dosage to an effective level.

One of the most common shortcomings in treating insomniac patients with antidepressant drugs is a failure to obtain an adequate therapeutic dosage level. Usually this results from the physician confusing the sedative side effects of these drugs with their antidepressant effects. Since the sedative effect is immediate and occurs with small doses, using this effect as the end point will most likely result in an inadequate dosage level.

In treating the elderly patient, the physician should be alert for possible paradoxical drug responses and drug intoxication. Many of the sedative-hypnotic drugs have been reported to cause occasional paradoxical drug reactions including agitation and extreme emotional lability in the elderly patient. This effect probably represents a disinhibition reaction and increasing the dose of the drug is contraindicated. Drug intoxication can occur easily in the elderly, since many drugs are metabolized more slowly in these patients. O'Malley et al. (1971) found that the half life of phenylbutazone and antipyrene was 78 percent longer in elderly females than in younger controls. Frequently, the combination of slowed metabolism and the effects of other drugs present can cause blood levels of a compound to reach toxic levels at relatively low dosages.

SUMMARY

We have summarized a number of ways in which sleep laboratory studies have contributed to our understanding of the aging process.

1. They have provided objective and precise techniques for determining not only how much sleep the elderly obtain, but also what type of sleep, i.e., specific sleep stages.

2. These studies have also provided a means for determining the frequency of dream recall in the elderly as well as the content of the recall.

3. The relation between penile erections in the male, and the REM cycle provides another means for assessing sexual capacity in the elderly, i.e., in determining frequency and amount of nocturnal erection.

4. Insomnia is a major complaint of the elderly. The sleep laboratory and related studies provide investigators with better objective means of evaluating and treating this common sleep disorder.

REFERENCES

Agnew, H. W., Webb, W. B., and Williams, R. L. (1966). Psychophysiology 2, 263.
Altshuler, K. A., Barad, M., and Goldfarb, A. I. (1963). Arch. Gen. Psychiat. 8, 33.
Aserinsky, E., and Kleitman, N. (1953). Science 118, 273.
Barad, M., Altshuler, K. A., and Goldfarb, A. I. (1961). Arch. Gen. Psychiat. 4, 419.
Dement, W. C., and Kleitman, N. (1957). Electroencephalog. Clin. Neurophysiol. 9, 673.
Dement, W. C., and Wolpert, E. A. (1958). J. Exp. Psychol. 55, 543.
Feinberg, I. (1969). In "Sleep Physiology and Pathology" (A. Kales, ed.), pp. 39-52, Lippincott, Philadelphia.
Feinberg, I., Koresko, R. L., and Heller, N. (1967). J. Psychiat. Res. 5, 107.
Fisher, C., Gross, J., and Zuch, J. (1965). Arch. Gen. Psychiat. 12, 29.
Goodenough, D. R., Shapiro, A., Holden, M., and Steinschriber, R. (1959). J. Abnorm. Soc. Psychol. 59, 295.
Kahn, E., and Fisher, C. (1967). "Dream Recall and Sleep Parameters of the Healthy Aged". Presented at the 7th Annual Meeting of the Association for the Psychophysiological Study of Sleep. Santa Monica.
Kahn, E., and Fisher, C. (1969a). J. Nervous Mental Disease 148, 477.
Kahn, E., and Fisher, C. (1969b). J. Gen. Psychiat. 2, 181.
Kales, A. (1968). Ann. Intern. Med. 68, 1078.
Kales, A., and Kales, J. D. (1972). In "The Relevance of Sleep Research to Clinical Practice" (G. Usdin, ed.), pp. 61-94, Brunner/Mazel, New York.
Kales, A., and Kales, J. D. (1974). New Engl. J. Med. 290, 478.
Kales, A., Wilson, T., Kales, J. D., Jacobson, A., Paulson, M. J., Kollar, E., and Walter, R. D. (1967). J. Am. Geriat. Soc. 15, 405.

Kales, A., Kales, J. D., and Bixler, E. O. (1974a). *Psychiat. Ann.* 4, 28.

Kales, A., Bixler, E. O., and Kales, J. D. (1974b). *In* "Advances in Sleep Research" (E. Weitzman, ed.), pp. 391-415, Spectrum Publications, Inc., Flushing, New York.

Karacan, I., Goodenough. D. R., Shapiro, A., and Starker, S. (1966). *Arch. Gen. Psychiat.* 15, 183.

O'Malley, K., Crooks, J., Duke, E., and Stevenson, I. H. (1971). *Brit. Med. J.* 3, 607.

Parmalee, A. H., Jr., Wenner, W. H., Akiyama, Y., Schultz, M., and Stern, E. (1967). *Develop. Med. Child Neurol.* 9, 70.

Rechtschaffen, A., and Kales, A. (eds.) (1968). A Manual of Standardized Terminology, Techniques and Scoring for Sleep Stages of Human Subjects. (NIH Publication No. 204), Government Printing Office, Washington, D. C.

Rechtschaffen, A., Vogel, G., and Shaikun, G. (1963). *Arch. Gen. Psychiat.* 9, 536.

Rechtschaffen, A., Hauri, V., and Zeitlin, M. (1966). *Percept. Mot. Skills* 22, 927.

Roffwarg, H. P., Dement, W. C., and Fisher, C. (1964). *In* "Problems of Sleep and Dream in Children: Monographs on Child Psychiatry" (E. Harms, ed.), pp. 60-72, Pergamon Press, New York.

Webb, W. B. (1970). *Intern. Psychiat. Clin.* 7, 29.

Weisz, R. (1969). "Dreams of the Aged; An EEG Study". Presented at the 9th Annual Meeting of the Association for the Psychological Study of Sleep. Boston.

SEXUAL INADEQUACY IN THE ELDERLY

Ruth B. Weg, Ph.D.

Department of Biology
Andrus Gerontology Center
University of Southern California
Los Angeles, California

Background

From a poem by Eve Merriam (1972) -- a fiercely alive old woman -- yet close to death -- in a hospital gown -- standing alone with a shopping bag, carrying all her life's possessions, and talking "A Conversation Against Death":

"You think I couldn't make you a good lover still?
You're crazy if you don't think so.
I could make you miserable with anyone else.
You would close your eyes with those tame tootsies
And dream about me, plead for me . . . . "

But the society at large still equates sexual inadequacy with aging. Oriented to sex for the young, the middle-aged and aged are not expected to be sexually active and fully functional. Desire has been cooled by the years, and if still simmering, the frail old are not capable of love making. More importantly, it may even be hazardous. Many older persons, vulnerable for many reasons, fulfill this prophecy and submit to the myth of the "sexless non-person".
All of us are still the recipients of the legacy from earlier cross-sectional studies which tested ill, institutionalized elderly with college youth and, predictably, found the older person with marginal percentages of the capacities of youth. But, recently, there has been the realization that the nature of aging changes can best be illuminated via longitudinal studies. Through Dr. Nathan Shock's work (1970, 1974) and the NIH 11-year longitudinal study of healthy elderly men (Birren et al., 1963, 1974; Graneck, 1971), it is now generally accepted that the decrements of function, systems and tissues are gradual and not as widespread as suggested in

the earlier research. These changes of capacity in muscle strength and tone, in skin elasticity, in visual acuity, in intellectual function, in cardiovascular activity, and in reproductive capacity are, in general, accommodated by the body and by the person.

Although most older persons accept the notion that climbing a mountain may no longer be possible, changes in the reproductive system take on an oppressive aura for most -- bring concern for success or failure as a sexual partner -- and frequently create a frightening ego-damaging trauma. Reproductive decline appears to usher in the end of all of productive life -- and the culture still largely equates sexual performance with manliness or womanliness. Any loss or dysfunction in this capacity, therefore, is construed as a step closer to death, and conjures up the terrible image of sexuality.

Primitive and modern man alike have been in search of rejuvenation and immortality. There has been and still is related to this search the equating of sex with death and/or life, especially long life. Exploration has spanned the gamut from magic and sorcery with potions and elixirs through folklore remedies of plant and animal tissues to the claims for Gerovital (Aslan, 1972). Most frequently, the measure of youth and the potential for immortality were sexual capacity and performance (Trimmer, 1970). In the biblical days of King David of Israel, the ministrations and body warmth of a young virgin was the final treatment to help revive the aging, ill king. Throughout history, aging males have sought aphrodisiacs or sex stimulants to extend the "manliness" of sexual potency. First recorded recipes were allegedly found on a Babylonian cuneiform tablet, 800 B.C. In China, between 350 and 250 B.C., prevailing Taoist prolongevitism led to elaborate techniques to augment and conserve body "essence" or semen (Gruman, 1966). Dr. E. Steinach, in 1920, picked up on this concept and suggested that tying off sperm ducts (vas deferens) would provide an internal accumulation of sex hormones and make the individual young again (Trimmer, 1970).

Plants such as orchids, sweet potatoes, mandrake, and countless others had been recommended earlier as sexual rejuvenants (Trimmer, 1970). Animal products for rejuvenation, including the use of partridge brains and Chinese bird nest soup, reach a peak with the use of sex glands and/or their extracts by Dr. Brown-Séquard, a French physician and scientist. Using himself as the experimental animal in 1889, he injected the extracts from testes of guinea pigs. However, his Parisian colleagues scoffed at his claim that three injections had turned the clock back 30 years. After World War I, the insertion of slices of chimpanzee testes in the bursae of male patients ushered in the vogue of " monkey gland" grafting as rejuvenation treatment. Indeed, the sex hormone and cell therapy of today had their experimental origins back in the 19th Century (Guillerme, 1963).

Sexuality and the Whole Person

The importance of sex and sexuality for society is obvious; procreation insures the continuance of the human race. Sexual differentiation is the substrate for relationships between man and woman and the structural patterns of family. Expression of sexuality is a composite of prenatal developmental and postnatal learning experiences superimposed on a definite, inherent sexuality. It is therefore inescapable that in human sexuality, as in so many other aspects of behavior, people are extremely flexible and behaviors cover a wide spectrum.

The sexual hormones involved in the development of reproductive structure and function from conception through old age stimulate sexual attraction and activity. These same hormones affect other developmental processes such as protein synthesis, salt and water balance, bone growth and resorption, cardiovascular function and possibly the immune surveillance mechanisms. Most human beings are completely provided with the natural, biologic equipment for reproduction and sexual interactions. However, human sexuality is more than the reproductive system, hormones, and sexual intercourse; it connotes the capacity for involvement in all of life that grows from the fact that there are two sexes.

The total personality participates in the complexities of sexual behavior and is not separable in practice from the anatomy and physiology involved. For the individual, the acts of intimacy and warmth associated with sexuality have a significance beyond the pleasurable release of sexual tension. As a reaffirmation of the connection with other of life's functions, it is an important assertion and commitment of self. Many psychologists and psychiatrists see some danger in the preoccupation with sexual technique and the resulting depersonalization of sex. Dr. Rollo May has stated, "Sex becomes a meaningless aside, a 'cul-de'sac' when looked upon as an isolated human function" (Gorney and Cox, 1973).

Sexuality in Old Age

Older men are often arbitrarily seen by public and professionals alike as somehow sexually impaired (Masters and

Johnson, 1970). The apprehension of becoming old is co-mingled with fear of loss of sexual adequacy and is a common preoccupation of the man of middle and later years. Nevertheless, men appear to fare somewhat better than women. Witness the plaudits for older men who remain sexually involved at whatever level, e.g., a late marriage is seen as a sign of vitality. There is a widespread acceptance of the 50-year old man who chooses a new friend or wife of 28. This liasion between a young woman and a man who could be her father is considered normal. Unfortunately, only a minority of older men are in a position to have this choice. When status, job, and power have been left behind, the identification of male vigor with achievement is difficult. Loss of confidence and depreciating self-image may lead to difficulty, if not impotence in sexual relations.

"That old women are repulsive is one of the most profound esthetic and erotic feelings in our culture" (Sontag, 1972). Many people are revolted by the thought of an old woman making love with a young man. An analytical view identifies the youth as a victim of the oedipal complex. Marriage of an older woman to a younger man is a break with a fierce taboo. The kindest evaluation of older women assigns them too frequently to yet a third sex -- the neuters of society. A developmental cycle is completed from "young and sexy" to "mature and exciting" and finally from 50 on into the anonymity of the sexually unseen (Butler and Lewis, 1973). Yet, in some countries, the older wife and the younger husband marriage is increasing. In West Germany, in 1973, about 70,000 such marriages took place; in Britain, it is increasing 10-fold in recent years; in Sweden, 12-fold (Butler, 1975).

<u>Role of Sex and Sexuality in Later Life</u>

The need for intimacy and love, as with other human needs for dignity, self concept, involvement, and intellectual growth, begins very early in the human baby and continues all through life. These needs and wants are not banished from human personality and behavior in the middle or late years, at 50 or 65. On the contrary, the reality of an "intimate other" may be more critical in these older years when life space has diminished and meaningful relationships are fewer, as friends and relatives move away or die (Lowenthal and Berkman <u>et al</u>., 1967). Roles as citizen, worker, and active parent may be lost or less structured as power and influence slowly disappear. Most recently, an article suggested that the expression of the sensual and sexual needs of the aged could be considered an important deterrent to suicide (Leviton, 1973).

There is increased agreement among those who study sexual responses among older people, that sex and sexuality can provide important psychological and physiological outlets as the years advance. The late psychologist, Dr. Lawrence Frank (1961), identified the opportunity for sexual relations as an important primary source of psychological reinforcement for some older people. This, he suggested, was particularly true for men at a time when they face loss of the prestige and self-confidence that accompanies their narrowing work world. For women, the need becomes critical when they fear a diminution of attractiveness and desirability following menopause. "What people need and want is intimacy and authentic love" (May, 1969).

Studies, beginning with the now classic works of Kinsey (1948, 1953) on sexual behavior in the human male and female, and continuing with the significant work of Masters and Johnson (1966, 1970) and others (Pfeiffer and Davis, 1972) have amply documented that sexual interest and activity may persist through the ninth decade of life -- even after the ninth decade of life. With marital partners aged 60-74, 60% remain sexually active and about 30% after 75 (Busse, 1973). While it is true that sexual interest and activity decrease with the advancing years, cessation is most often found to be a function of decline of physical health of one or both of the partners. Upon comparison of the sex urge in youth and old age, there remains a remarkable constancy of sexual drives throughout life. Older men are generally more active than women, but this difference may be more apparent than real. Women who are old today formed their attitudes and practices related to sex activity during an earlier Victorian period. Mores and morality up to now have dictated the woman's primary sexual role is procreative, and interest in sex beyond that, improper. Today, there are more older women than men and most older women are widowed. Between 65 and 74 years, women outnumber men 130/100. This ratio climbs to 166 women to 100 men after 75 years (Brotman, 1973, 1974). The absence of a capable, socially sanctioned mate is a forceful, inhibiting factor (Pfeiffer and Davis, 1972).

Sexuality for Older Men and Women: Behavior and Physiology

Loss of sexual vigor should be no greater than loss of other physical capabilities (Rubin, 1965; Masters and Johnson, 1970). Rather, impotency before advanced age (between 80 and 90 years) often appears to be a function of psychological problems rather than physical incapacities. The misconception that loss of fertility associated with the decrease in sexual hormones is causally related to depressed libido and basic competence is easily refuted by data from clinical evidence (Masters and Johnson, 1970; Pfeiffer and Davis, 1972). Age does not necessarily alter performance nor does it eliminate the quality of satisfaction and pleasure of sexual gratification (Greenblatt and Leng, 1972).

Longitudinal studies provide the most useful information about changes with time of an individual's capacities. Such an investigation over a six-year period was reported by the Duke University Center for the Study of Aging and Human Development (Pfeiffer and Davis, 1972). Primarily white, middle, and upper class men and women were tested and interviewed for a two-day period at appropriate intervals. A larger number of variables influenced current sexual behavior of men as compared with women. Increased age, antihypertensive drugs, declining health, and anxiety over the examination had a measurable negative effect. Past enjoyment, interest and frequency, three indicators of early sexual life function, correlated positively with present interests and activity among men and women. For the older women, however, current interest and activity were more dependent upon marital status. This confirmed previous observations that among elderly women today, the presence of an interested, able mate is not always enough. Optimally, he also needs to be her marriage partner. Cessation of sexual relations was reported by 14% of the males and 40% of the females. Women attribute cessation to mates and the men confirmed this statement. This reemphasizes earlier findings that the pattern of marital coitus (particularly among the middle-aged and aged) is typically controlled by male desire and his aging, rather than by the wife's loss of interest or capacity. In their controversial report on an 11-year scientific inquiry into physiology of sex among nearly 800 men and women, Masters and Johnson added a qualifying note to the measured and observed active involvement in sexuality: with age there was a decrease in the intensity and rapidity of response (Masters and Johnson, 1970). Commonalities between men and women as reproductive and sexual human beings exist, but are often ignored. Changes in hormones during the climacteric affect older men and women alike in alteration of sleep patterns, weight gain, receding hair growth, loss of hair color and genital tissues. Children know sexuality as a generalized body response, and in "the primary sexual response of the adult male and female, there is no differentiation between man and woman". . . the basic qualities of orgasm are "the same for male and female" (Roszak, 1969). However, it is equally useful to look at men and women separately for the particular physiological changes and especially as they bring these capacities into meaningful relationships.

The Male: Anatomy and Physiology

As with other aspects of normal aging, reduced function does not mean absence of capacity. The reproductive system of the man is measurably different in form and function at ages 60 to 80 from what it was at 20, 30, and 50 years of age. In one study, one-half of the men aged 75 to 92 reported continued sexual intercourse (Rubin, 1964). Other investigations revealed the average frequency of coitus for the majority of men over 65 is four times per month. Dr. Rutherford (1971) indicated that couples in their 50's have coitus 1.8 times per week on the average, in contrast to 4.8 times per week of young marrieds -- by the 60's the frequency is 1.3 times per week. Masturbation is a recurrent practice among 25% of them (Tarail, 1962).

Physical Changes

In men, male hormone (testosterone) production continues into old age. Although testosterone is available at a higher level for a longer period than estrogen is in women, the concentration is increasingly inadequate and does affect the genital tissues. A gradual decline in sex energy, muscle strength, and number of viable sperm result from this steroid depletion. The testes become smaller and less firm; testicular tubules thicken and begin a degenerative process which finally inhibits the production of sperm. As the prostate gland enlarges, its contractions become weaker. There is a reduction in volume and viscosity of seminal fluid so that the force of ejaculation decreases. No one of these changes are major, but together they are responsible for some real and apparent changes in the total expression of sexuality.

The Female: Anatomy and Physiology

Physiologically, the older woman need experience little sexual difficulty. If moderately good health, a positive attitude toward sex, and an available, effective sexual partner prevail, sexual activity can extend until the very late years (until 90). Nevertheless, certain myths and stereotypes that have surrounded the menopause persist in aging, *i.e.*, the end to sexual desire and attractiveness culminating in defeminization, the inevitability of depression, involutional melancholia and even insanity. These myths have been repeatedly refuted by physicians, psychologists, psychiatrists; practitioners, and researchers alike (Deutsch, 1945; Benedek, 1959; Neugarten, 1968; Masters and Johnson, 1970). Masters and Johnson as well as others feel "There is no time limit drawn by advancing years to female sexuality" (Masters and Johnson, 1966). They found significant sexual capacity and effective sexual performance among 61 menopausal and postmenopausal women, 40 - 78 years (Masters and Johnson, 1970).

However, cultural expectations and early role models compounded by ignorance may lead to severe psychological reactions. In a society where so much is measured by the yardstick of youth, its unlined beauty, vigor and performance, anxieties mount over attractiveness, the empty nest, and the evaluation of career, community involvement, and marriage.

There is no inevitability about major physical or psychological crises pre-, during, or postmenopause. Statistical morbidity and mortality data demonstrate that long years of good health remain (Brotman, 1973). Each female will live through a highly individualized pattern of menopause and postmenopause. Freed from fear of pregnancy and care of children, some may seek new sexual partners with interest, while others look forward to the end of their sexual involvement which may have provided limited pleasure and gratification.

The Climacteric

This total period begins when many women are in their forties and ordinarily may span 20 - 30 years. It is characterized by a sequence of phases: reduced fertility; irregular or absent menses; blood vessel instability and anatomical atrophy. The phases will vary in degree and extent depending upon the individual's rate of change.

(1) A decrease in likelihood of pregnancy develops. The remaining follicles are those that are least susceptible to stimulation by pituitary gonadotropins.

(2) Estrogen concentration and activity decrease in proportion to the decrease in follicular maturation, and decreased corpora lutea formation. This reduced amount of estrogen is insufficient to stimulate uterine lining to the former premenstrual proliferated state. Secondary sex characteristics and other estrogen-related metabolic processes (protein synthesis, bone formation, salt and water balance, reciprocal hormonal interaction

with other glands) are maintained at a reasonably homeostatic level for some time (often until late 60's).

(3) Menopause. During the two-to-three year period of irregular menses prior to total cessation of menstruation, there may be irregular bleeding which is usually correctable by dilation and curettage, if necessary. Statistics indicate 25 - 30% of postmenopausal bleeding may be due to malignancy, but between 70 - 75% of all bleeding will cease without medical or surgical intervention. Other complaints that may be noted during this period include palpitation, irritability, anxiety, depression, loss of appetite, insomnia and headache. They are relatively infrequent and do not involve enough women to be called "characteristic of menopause".

(4) Upon follicle exhaustion, the primary estrogen source is gone. Although the adrenal synthesizes and releases hormones that are metabolized to female sex hormones, progressive diminution may lead to loss of support to vascular and genital tissues. For some women, a common transitory discomfort is the "hot flash", experienced as the result of a troublesome, periodic dilation of small blood vessels. The "flash" involves heat, sweat, and patchy redness starting on the chest and extending to neck and face. It is equally significant that many women complete the climacteric and never experience the "flash".

There is a difference of opinion concerning the etiology of the vascular instability, but it may be due to the increased secretion of pituitary gonadotropin without the moderating, reciprocal effect of the estrogen/progesterone.

(5) Finally, between the ages of 60 - 70 years, the continued sex steroid "starvation" results in atrophy of the uterus, vagina, and involution of related genital tissues. Mild regression of secondary sexual characteristics may occur:

- Skin elasticity decreases; glandular tissue and tone diminish causing ligaments to relax so that breast and other area contours are less firm.

- There is a loss of vulvar substance, the mons flattens and major labia are less full.

- Vaginal mucosa thins and decreases in length with disappearance of the rugal pattern. Estrogen deficient vaginitis may be present.

- Cervix, corpus uterus, and ovaries shrink at times to prepubertal size.

- There is a modest reduction in the size of the clitoris, the minor labial covering or hood atrophies along with the mons fatty tissue. For the clitoris, however, there is "no objective evidence to date to suggest any appreciable loss in sensate focus" (Masters and Johnson, 1970).

- Bartholin glands that lubricate the vagina may decrease with age.

- Portions of the urinary tract, the urethra and bladder frequently suffer similar atrophy.

(6) Possible pathology. The sex steroid starvation has frequently been linked to some of the chronic diseases associated with aging. Specific diseases have been linked to estrogen deficiency. There is a statistical rise in atherosclerotic changes in the coronary blood vessels in postmenopausal women and in younger women with removal of ovaries (Davis et al., 1961; Higano et al., 1963). Moreover, estrogen-treated ovariectomized women experience fewer coronary accidents. However, the cause and effect is not quite that singular or direct. Although the etiology of atherosclerosis and any consequent coronary accidents are not clear, female sex hormones seem to be part of the enzymatic machinery in the metabolism of fats and proteins. Beyond that, heredity, total diet, exercise, and stressful life-style have also been implicated (Selye, 1970, 1973; Newton and Morgan, 1968).

Osteoporosis, identified as osteopenia by Dr. Garn, is the leaking out of calcium, with a measurable loss of bone mass which leads to diminished height, instability in maintenance of normal posture, ease of fracture, and often acute pain. Some estrogen-treated women and men are stabilized, others do not respond (Bartter, 1973). There is research that indicates exercise and life-long dietary habits may be more important than estrogen in maintenance of bone structure (Lutwak, 1969). Good results have been reported with greater calcium intake which increases retention of protein and activation of osteoblasts. Another factor, genetic in origin, may be the porosity of the bone. It is conceivable that those with more porous bones may be more susceptible to any estrogen-primed alteration in calcium metabolism. Finally, if estrogen were solely responsible, estrogen therapy should inhibit and even reverse the progress of osteoporosis in men. Such is not the case. Studies are then equivocal and would require continued pursuit of a more exact molecular mechanism that would enable a predictive or preventive therapy.

As Sexual Partners

There is a recognizable difference in sexual responsiveness and activity with age. At the Reproduction Biology Research Foundation in St. Louis, Masters and Johnson (1970), using clinical observations and interviews, have documented, for the first time, the significant changes with age in the physiology of the sex act.

Although most males over 60 engage in intercourse once or twice a week, the capacity to enjoy sex more frequently is probably greater than that number indicates and depends upon appropriate stimulation to erection. Natural delays in achieving erection are accompanied by the capacity to maintain the erection longer without reaching orgasm. This reduction in ejaculatory demand is appropriate to the slower excitation response in the older woman, and serves to enhance the possibility of increased arousal and orgasm to the greater satisfaction of both.

Other factors not directly related to physiological capacities or health may also modify the sexual patterns of older men (either reduction of sexual activity or increase of extramarital sex) may relate more to the quality of the relationship with mate, *e.g.*, a marriage partner of 30 years is often cited as a reasonable basis of boredom for the male.

Frequency of intercourse, intensity of sensation, speed of attaining erection, and force of ejaculation are all reduced. To a greater or lesser degree (a function of individual differences) each of the four phases of intercourse depart from the youthful pattern (Masters and Johnson, 1966, 1970).

(1) Excitement phase. Excitement builds more slowly. Intensity and duration of the sex flush and involuntary spasms are diminished. Erection, longer to attain, has stimulated little testicular elevation or scrotum vasocongestion.

(2) Plateau phase. The plateau phase usually lasts longer than during youth, with minimal vascular engorgement of testes. Increase in penile circumference is marked by absence or reduction of pre-ejaculatory fluid emission.

(3) Orgasmic phase. In older men, the orgasmic phase is usually of shorter duration and may have a reduced or totally missing first stage or ejaculatory demand. In most younger males, the entire ejaculatory process is divided into two well recognized stages: the first ejaculatory inevitability is brief (2 - 4 seconds) in which control is very difficult; the second marks the expulsion of the seminal fluid bolus through the full length of the penis and may be complete within one or two contractions in older men, as contrasted with four or more at a younger age.

(4) Resolution phase. In the older man, the loss of erection and return of the penis to a flaccid state may take a few seconds compared to youth's minutes or hours. The subsequent refractory period in the aging male may be extended from the two minutes of the younger male to 12 - 24 hours.

As with older men, both neuronal (decrease in rate of responsivity) and hormonal (steroid starvation) factors combine to affect the recognizable changes in anatomy and function of older women as sexual partners.

The act of coitus may prove unsatisfying and even painful to some postmenopausal women. The thinning vaginal walls and decreased lubrication may make penetration difficult. If cracking of vaginal walls has occurred, there may be some bleeding and pain. Under hormonal deprivation, uterine contractions, as part of the female orgasm, may also cause pain. Burning and frequency of urination after intercourse may also occur since the atrophic bladder and urethra are more susceptible to irritation and not as protected by the thinning vagina. With advancing years, the intensity of physiological response to effective stimulation are decreased through all four phases of the cycle (Masters and Johnson, 1966, 1970).

(1) Excitement phase. Lubrication time is increased from a matter of 15 - 30 seconds to as much as five minutes. This is comparable to the involution of the aging male in whom erective delay is a natural fact of aging. The purplish hue of vasocongestion in the younger

woman has changed to pink in the older woman.

(2) Plateau phase. Involuntary uterine elevation is reduced. There is a lack of the deep sex skin coloration in the minor labia, so predictive of impending orgasm. The major labia do not elevate and flatten against the perineum as in younger women, and may hang limply in folds around the vaginal opening. The clitoral response includes the elevation and flattening on the anterior border of the symphysis, similar to that in younger women.

(3) Orgasmic phase. Duration of orgasm is considerably reduced between the ages of 50 to 70 years. Uterine contractibility from fundus to midzone to lower segment may be similar to that of younger women, but rather than rhythmic, may be spastic and pain-inducing. The contractions are fewer, from 3 - 5 to as low as 1 or 2. Vaginal orgasmic platform of outer one-third is still initiated within eight second intervals, but contractions are reduced from 8 - 12 to 4 - 5 times.

(4) Resolution phase. Rapid resolution, as with older men, is characteristic of female sex steroid imbalance. Pelvic viscera return to prestimulatory state; uterus to nonelevated position, and the moderately expanded vaginal canal collapses. If any minor labia color change is present, it is faint and its disappearance is initiated even before orgasm is reached.

These normal anatomical and physiological modulations of the female reproductive system are not experienced either in part or all, by every woman at the same time. Moreover, these changes do not alter the fact that in most reports, since Kinsey *et al*. (1953), there is no falling off in sexual arousability with rising age. In fact, frequently there is an increase. The inference for a lifetime of sexuality is clear from the fact that, for women, regularity of sexual stimulation and activity will overcome the effect of sex steroid inadequacy or starvation. Reportedly, the pattern of masturbatory release of sexual tension is increased in women after menopause through the 6th and 7th decade, and in men after the age of 65.

The functional separation of fertility and libido is best revealed in the high level of sexual desire and activity reported by women after hysterectomy (Post, 1967). Menopausal and postmenopausal women maintain the multiorgasmic capacity of their younger years (Kinsey et al., 1953; Masters and Johnson, 1970; Roszak, 1969).

Nevertheless, menopausal and older women, who have chosen to use their energies for homemaking and mothering, may experience greater difficulty coping with the symptoms of these midlife physiological changes (Neugarten, 1968; Rutherford and Rutherford, 1966). Those women who have been able to combine the homemaker and worker roles (outside the home) would appear to be largely free of most of the psychological and physical responses that were said to be inevitable (Glass and Kase, 1970; Gorney and Cox, 1973).

Bases for Dysfunction

If, indeed, the normal aging of the reproductive system leaves older men and women with active interest and capacity -- what are the factors that contribute to the dysfunctional, sexless, impotent image of those over 65? They tend to be the same factors that would affect sexuality and the whole person at any age: disease and surgery of the urogenital system, other systemic diseases, drug abuse, excessive work with consequent fatigue, excessive eating and alcoholism, and lastly, closely interlaced with the aforementioned and societal attitudes -- emotional disturbance.

Declining level of general health and current practice in treatment of the complaints of older patients have lead to widespread drug abuse (Townsend, 1971; Lamy and Kitler, 1971). Alcohol, marijuana and tranquilizers (e.g. chlorpromazine, librium, mellaril, reserpine) weaken erection and delay ejaculation. Unabated use may lead to impotency. Depression, fear of failure, anemia, diabetes, fatigue, malnutrition, and a variety of metabolic abnormalities at any stage of life, if untreated, may inhibit desire, abort arousal and sexual climax, and logically influence the entire physical and affective quality of living. Overeating and consequent obesity may substitute for sexual desire, have serious consequences for cardiovascular health, and be particularly damaging for self image.

With advancing age, there is the increased possibility of one or more chronic diseases which alone or in combination, may have secondary physiological effects on the reproductive system and modify sexual expression, either directly or indirectly. The major source of difficulty is fear on the part of the older person that any sexual involvement will exacerbate an illness, even lead to death (Masters and Johnson, 1970; Rubin, 1966a, b).

Coronary Disease

During sexual intercourse, heart rate, blood pressure, and oxygen consumption increase at levels comparable to moderate rather than strenuous exercise. As such, sexual activity rather than a threat to health may be both therapeutic and preventive, e.g., there is an increase in adrenal corticoids which relieves some of the symptoms of arthritis; the sense of well-being reduces physical and emotional tensions. For the sake of an estimate, of 1% sudden coronary death during or after intercourse (Butler and Lewis, 1973), the unique benefits of human warmth and sexuality are lost to many. In a study of 91 middle-aged, middle class men, it was found that sexual activity was resumed on an average of 13.7 weeks after coronary accident, occurring earlier in previously sexually more active people (Hellerstein and Friedman, 1970). There is the repeated suggestion that sexual past history and experience are more significant as determinants than any other factor. Only extreme coronary pathology would appear to call for abstinence. As in youth, pain, malaise, and fear effectively suppress libido and magnify the aging and already declining capacity.

Hypertension

In a particular study in Australia, Laver (1974) found that sexual activity in severely hypertensive males is often absent or at least decreased. Many of the patients assign the decrease in sexual potency to their drug therapy. The nature of their sexual dysfunction included erectile ability, libido, and ejaculation. Loss of erectile ability, despite the presence of libido and sexual arousal, may best be explained on a peripheral pharmacological basis -- and is the single most common complaint attributable to therapy. Loss of libido may result from the central sedative effect possessed by many of the drugs similar in nature to that seen with phenothiazines. Failure of ejaculation is rare in the presence of ability to maintain an erection in this study. All patients with any difficulty were quite certain, whatever cause will eventually be identified, that the "pills" they were taking to treat the hypertension were interfering with their sexual potency. Another barrier to sexual activity is the characteristic belief of most hypertensive patients (and shared by many individuals with ischemic heart disease) that, in view of their illness, sexual activity was dangerous. The implications are clear: careful testing of new hypertensive drugs needs to consider side effects, particularly related to sexual activity and adequate sex education and counseling for those individuals with coronary involvement.

Diabetes

Sexual dysfunction is a common accompaniment of diabetes in men and women despite continued libido. In women, there is reported difficulty in vaginal lubrication although vaginal mucosa and cytology indicate adequate estrogen. No specific etiology could be implicated and it was generally identified as secondary orgasmic dysfunction (Kolodny et al., 1974). Numerous investigators have suggested that about 50% of diabetic males with organic impotence are unable to masturbate or stimulate erection in any way. The basic etiology of the impotence is not at all definitive and it is still an area for research and discussion.

Although low testosterone levels have been implicated by some studies, more verification is needed. Frequently, concentration is within normal range (Kolodny et al., 1974). Hormone therapy (testosterone alone or in common with chorionic gonadotropin) has not been successful in treating diabetes-related impotence. There are possible adverse effects from testosterone therapy, i.e., sodium retention, hepatic dysfunction, prostatic hypertrophy, and potential increase in libido while erectile dysfunction remains. This last side effect may, in fact, further frustrate and disturb the patient whose libido was sufficient in any case.

Large vessel disease (as vascular complications in diabetes; Leriche Syndrome), may bring about impotence, perhaps as a secondary consequence to microvascular changes. More recent emphasis in impotence associated with diabetes has been on a neurological basis -- libido may decrease and be lost, a process taking several months to a year. As an example, polsters, valve-like structures containing smooth muscle, have been described near the corpora cavernosa and are under control of the autonomic nervous system. Poor neural transmission may disturb the steady increased blood inflow to the erectile tissues (H.D. Weiss, 1972). More recently, Faerman et al. (1973) found biological evidence of autonomic neuropathy in neural fibers of corpora cavernosa.

Other kinds of sexual dysfunction may further complicate diabetes, including retrograde ejaculation and premature ejaculation. In view of a lack of effective therapy for such dysfunction, it is critical that the physician identify the causes of impotence, and they are numerous.

Potency

With the current emphasis on sexual adequacy, it may become important to define sexual potency, as follows: "ability to activate psyche or (emotional) desire for sexual intercourse into penile erection adequate for coitus and to achieve gratification (usually ejaculation) during the sexual act" (Finkle and Moyers, 1960). In describing potency after prostatectomy, they added this condition should have been met within one year following the surgery in order to be considered potent. Potency may be examined according to its probable origin:

(1) Erective difficulty may be a result of drug therapy caused by drugs such as antidepressants, antihypertensives, estrogens, tranquilizers. Alcohol is statistically the most frequent factor in the development of impotence.

(2) Impotence of organic origin is most often related to diabetes. The onset is slow (over a period of 6 months to a year), libido is also reduced and, as earlier mentioned, there is an inability to masturbate or stimulate erection in any way. Impotence following prostatectomy usually has a much more abrupt onset, characterized by a complete lack of ability to attain morning erections or masturbate although libido may be considerable and shall be dealt with in greater detail below.

(3) A variety of factors such as stress, boredom, concern with job or career and other variables of psychogenic origin may lead to impotence. Such impotence is generally of abrupt onset and frequently reversible. Libido is low, and masturbation to orgasm ability is maintained. Often a change of partner alleviates the disorder. Depression and anxiety often accompany organic impotence, resulting in a psychologic overlay. Some women, who are now old, may suffer from sexual dysfunction related to frigidity or vaginismus, both of which may occur at any age and generally are psychogenic in origin.

(4) Surgery/urogenital system. Perhaps the most direct effects are those that derive from dysfunction or surgery of the urogential system. Pelvic surgery has signaled an end to effective sexual activity for large numbers of older men and women. Clinical data suggests that although prostatectomies and hysterectomies appear to depress desire and capacity for climax, they are not inevitable

physiological consequences of the surgery (Finkle and Moyers, 1960). The suggestion that emotion (fear of inadequacy, concern with the sexless image) was of greater importance than the surgery is reasonable. More than 80% of patients following prostatectomy, and 70% of women following hysterectomy retain potency and coital enjoyment (Patterson and Craig, 1963). Moreover, there are men and women who have low sex drives, and such surgery may be a welcome excuse for cessation. Loss of potency, however, is a common occurrence, and well-documented, following perineal exposure and removal of prostate. In recent investigations into suprapubic and transurethral surgery, of a total of 94 individuals, 80% experienced no significant change in sexual potency; 69% of 61 - 70 year olds retained potency (some reduced) one year after surgery, independent of age. One male over 80 experienced no change in sexual potency and frequency of intercourse was maintained at four to six times monthly. Retrograde ejaculation was frequent, however, and a disturbing consequence to prostatic surgery. Of an entire group of 76 patients, 81% reported retrograde ejaculation. It would appear that a thorough explanation to the patient is in order prior to surgery (Gold and Hotchkiss, 1969).

What can be done to maximize the remaining capacity?

(1) Masters has stated, "The disinclination of medical and behavioral professions to treat the aging population for sexual dysfunction has been a major disservice perpetrated by those professionals upon the general problem" (Masters, 1974). At the Reproductive Biology Research Foundation in St. Louis, they have had 50% success rate with older people, in returning them to satisfying sexual activity. This is a higher failure rate than they have with younger subjects. They attribute this to the length of time the problem has existed and not to the age of the patient.

(2) There are suggestions that sexual activity be undertaken early in the day, when energy levels and hormones may be at their highest.

(3) Many therapists are of the opinion that masturbation may not only be necessary for those persons without available partners, but may be a means for many to know and enjoy their bodies. Realistically, with the uneven ratio of 166 women to 100 men over 75, and 130/100

between 65 and 74, there are large numbers of partnerless older women. It has been suggested that masturbation helps preserve potency in men and maintain the Bartholin gland functioning in women. Further, it releases tensions, stimulates sexual appetite and thereby contributes to general well being. The acceptance of masturbation as a legitimate pleasuring of one's body may be difficult for those who are old today -- but may indeed be more possible for generations to come.

(4) Polygamy is also suggested as a way out for the preponderance of older women. However, this solution is not attractive to all, some of the reaction may be related to the cohort effect again.

(5) Other approaches emphasize:

- equalizing the life span of men and women through research;

- equalizing of sex roles to give women the same opportunities as men;

- encouragement of dating and marriage by older women with younger men;

- development of more lenient attitudes toward already existent homosexuality, and, finally,

- find ways to increase life span and vigor of men.

Summary

The interaction of stress, hormonal activity, and general health and aging may be explored by measurable criteria (Selye, 1970). It is common knowledge that ovulation may be inhibited by systemic illness as well as by strong emotional experience, *e.g.*, anguish, fear, anxiety and asexual stimuli such as noise of voices. Even an unexplainable or unrecognizable sound intrusion can cause the loss of erection. Clinical data has accumulated to suggest that thought and affect can be parents to physiological change in youth and aging (Osofsky and Seidenberg, 1970; Brod *et al.*, 1959; J.M. Weiss, 1972; Rahe *et al.*, 1970). These correlations between psyche and physiology reinforce the interdependence of all body systems and put into sharper focus the importance of societal attitudes and support for older persons.

As with all other organ systems, normal aging of the reproductive system brings decreased efficiency, increased time for responsivity and tissue changes of internal and external genitalia. There is no question of the decrease in fertility -- few people over 65 retain or require the drive for more progeny! Unlike other organ systems, the human reproductive apparatus has function beyond child bearing. It is integrated as a major means of interpersonal communication involving the warmth and satisfaction unique to body contact.

Among older people, the basic human needs for intimacy, love, achievement, and self-concept are at greater risk at a time of life that augers so many other losses -- of friends, relatives, job status, active parenting, and decision-making. Compounding the shrinking functional world, the older man and woman face society's image of "neuter" and non-person. Fiction had been elevated to fact, and myth to reality by constant repetition so that older people have accepted their "third sex" fate and professionals have acted accordingly.

With the increasing numbers of older, healthier, more aware persons (growing in greater proportion to younger groups) demands for their fair share of life's offerings, and capacity for living more fully have been activated. Longitudinal studies have belied the mythology. Sensitive, supportive response from professionals and the society will potentiate what capacities older persons retain, rather than concentrate on the deficiencies. Otherwise, an overemphasis of sexuality related primarily to technique and frequency of orgasm, without reference to other aspects of the person, may prove to be negative and frustrating.

Implications of all of the above are:

(1) that the helping professional join with gerontologists in calling for departments of geriatrics in nursing schools, medical schools, and hospitals (Libow et al., 1972; Burnside, 1973).

(2) that gynecological and other medical textbooks in use be evaluated and culled to delete the myths related to aging men and women (Scully and Bart, 1973); e.g., in most texts, men are said to set the sexual pace for marital coitus, but nowhere is the multiorgasmic nature of women mentioned.

(3) that sex education be instituted for middle and old age (as well as for youth) so that older people may understand and accommodate, to extend and use what capacities persist.

(4) that sexuality be appropriately seen as a function of commonalities and differences, thereby appreciating the quality of a relationship, focusing on the person, not a performance.

(5) that the need for affect and sexual expression (outside of intercourse) be recognized as essential to being and feeling alive; that they be nurtured especially in older people for the mental and physical well being that ensures.

(6) that continued effort be made in the society at large, for greater acceptance of alternate life styles that could ameliorate the alienation of those who are single, alone, and old.

(7) that although there may be no substitute for another person in the fulsome pleasure of sexual expression, masturbation may be a necessary outlet for sexual release and maintenance of genital tissue readiness.

(8) that serious consideration be given to replacement estrogen therapy for most middle-aged and older women as a viable alternative to psychotherapy and sedation in the prevention and/or treatment of the emotional and physiological changes that accompany middle and old age (Masters and Johnson, 1970; Schleyer-Saunders, 1971; Sheffery et al., 1969). Phenobarbital or mellaril will not alter the skeletal, genital, and muscular tissue changes. While psychotherapy may alleviate or prevent a serious depression, only estrogen replacement can affect the metabolic apparatus directly. The specter of cancer with hormone therapy hasn't developed as earlier anticipated (Rhoades, 1965; Glass and Kase, 1970). More than 90% of uterine cancers are in women over 40 years, and breast cancer also increases with age when estrogen stores are low: 1.8% before 30, 75% develop over 40 (Leis, 1967). Estrogen in combination with testosterone does retard the tissue changes and other physiological symptomology associated with the climacteric (Masters and Johnson, 1970); many of the common complaints can be completely avoided with replacement therapy (Rogers, 1969).

(9) that research and observation into sexual adequacy and behavior be accelerated as an important consideration in the psychophysiology of aging, and finally,

(10) that sexual dysfunction in the elderly (and in younger people as well) appears to be related, in large part, to the degree and kind of pathologies that develop with increasing age, since normal aging generally brings a slow decline but not impotence. Therefore, the research challenge includes:

- extended study of the pharmacology of drugs in use (and abuse) in older patients.

- the identification of mechanism and treatment for neuropathy and vascular changes in diabetes.

- the definitive etiology and prevention of atherosclerosis.

- the early elimination of hypertension and coronary accidents.

- some intensive research into sex steroid therapy for males comparable to the estrogen therapy for females.

In a recent publication, Robert Butler (1975) states that, as with other aspects of aging, "there is a developmental potential to sexuality". People can and do acquire "new insights and new levels of feeling during a lifetime of lovemaking". He suggests there are "two dominant languages of sex". The one more direct and explosive is that in which response has been measured, frequency counted, and outlets specified. A second experiential language of sex involves caressing, touching, and tenderness. Both languages may be "intuitively present or acquired in early life", and be sources of great pleasure and satisfaction to the individual. There is now ample demonstration that the old are physically capable of sex, it may be the old will be able to make the most of the second language to enrich the expression of sexuality.

Sex is not the same in age as in youth -- and love and sex vary throughout the course of life (Butler, 1975). Maurice Chevalier seemed to accept that concept with his own statement, "There are 10,000 ways of loving. The main thing is to choose the one that goes best with your age". Hopefully, the future looks to a change in the psychosocial ambience in the society -- toward aging as part of living and sexuality as part of aging.

REFERENCES

Aslan, A. (1972). *Proc. 9th Intern. Congr. Gerontol. Symposia Reports* 2, 115.
Bartter, F. C. (1973). *Perspectives Biol. Med.* 16, 215.
Benedek, T. (1959). *In* "American Handbook of Psychiatry" (S. Arieti, ed.), Basic Books, Inc., New York.
Birren, J. E., Butler, R. N., Greenhouse, S. W., Sokoloff, L., and Yarrow, M. R. (eds.) (1974). "Human Aging: A Biological and Behavioral Study". Dept. HEW Publ. No. (HSM) 71-9051, Washington, D. C. (formerly PHS Publ. No. 986, 1963).
Brod, I., Fencl, V., Hejl, V., and Jirka, J. (1959). *Clin. Sci.* 18, 269.
Brotman, H. B. (1973). *Perspectives in Aging* 11, 8.
Brotman, H. B. (1974). "Every Tenth American". Statement to U.S. Senate Special Committee on Aging.
Burnside, I. (1973). *Med. Arts Sci.* 27, 13.
Busse, E. (1973). *Psychiat. Spector* 9, 10.
Butler, R. (1975). *In* "The Later Years" (L. Brown, and E. Ellis, eds.), pp. 129-143, Publishing Sciences, Acton, Massachusetts.
Butler, R., and Lewis, M. (1973). "Aging and Mental Health". C. V. Mosby Company, St. Louis.
Davis, M. E., Jones, R. J., and Jarolem, C. (1961). *Am. J. Ob. Gyn.* 82, 1003.
Deutsch, H. (1945). "The Psychology of Women". Grune and Stratton, New York.
Faerman, I., Glocer, L., Fox, D., Jadzinsky, M. N., and Rapaport, M. (1973). *Excerpta Med.*, 8th Congress of the International Diabetes Federation, Brussels, Belgium.
Finkle, A., and Moyers, T. (1960). *J. Urol.* 84, 152.
Frank, L. (1961). "The Conduct of Sex". William Morrow, New York.
Glass, R., and Kase, N. (1970). "Women's Choice, A Guide to Contraception, Fertility, Abortion and Menopause". Basic Books, Inc., New York.
Gold, F., and Hotchkiss, R. (1969). *N.Y. State J. Med.* 69, 2987.
Gorney, S., and Cox, C. (1973). "After Forty". The Dial Press, New York.
Graneck, S. (1971). *In* "Human Aging II: An Eleven Year Biomedical and Behavior Study" (R. D. Patterson, ed.), Government Printing Office, Washington, D. C.
Greenblatt, R., and Leng, J. (1972). *J. Am. Geriat. Soc.* XX, 49.
Gruman, G. J. (1966). *Trans. Am. Phil. Soc.* 56, 45.

Guillerme, J. (1963). "Longevity". Walker and Company, New York.
Hellerstein, H., and Friedman, E. (1970). Scand. J. Rehab. Med. 2-3, 109.
Higano, N., Robinson, R., and Cohen, W. (1963). New Engl. J. Med. 268, 1123.
Kinsey, A. C., Pomeroy, W. B., and Martin, C. I. (1948). "Sexual Behavior in the Human Male". W. B. Saunders Company, Philadelphia.
Kinsey, A. C., Pomeroy, W. B., Martin, C. I., and Gebhard, P. H. (1953). "Sexual Behavior in the Human Female". W. B. Saunders Company, Philadelphia.
Kolodney, R., Kahn, C., Goldstein, H., and Barnett, D. (1974). Diabetes 23, 306.
Lamy, P., and Kitler, M. (1971). J. Am. Geriat. Soc. 19, 23.
Laver, M. C. (1974). Aust. N.Z.J. Med. 4, 29.
Leis, H. (1967). Med. World News 8, 63.
Leviton, D. (1973). Omega 4, 163.
Libow, L., Freeman, J., Harris, R., and Kobrynski, B. (1972). In "Educational Symposium", Gerontological Society Meetings, Puerto Rico.
Lowenthal, M., and Berkman, P. L. et al. (1967). "Aging and Mental Disorder in San Francisco". Jossey-Bass, San Francisco.
Lutwak, L. (1969). J. Am. Geriat. Soc. XVII, 115.
Masters, W. H. (1974). From remarks at a Lawyers' Wives' Meeting, Beverly Hills, Calif., May 3, 1974. Reported in the Los Angeles Times, May 4, 1974.
Masters, W. H., and Johnson, V. (1966). "Human Sexual Inadequacy". Little, Brown and Co., Boston.
Masters, W. H., and Johnson, V. (1970). "Human Sexual Response". Little, Brown and Co., Boston.
May, R. (1969). "Love and Will". W. W. Norton, New York.
Merriam, E. (1972). Ms Magazine 1, 80, September.
Neugarten, B. (ed.) (1968). "Middle Age and Aging". University of Chicago Press, Chicago.
Newton, H. F., and Morgan, D. B. (1968). Lancet 1, 232.
Osofsky, F., and Seidenberg, R. (1970). J. Ob. Gyn. 36, 611.
Patterson, R. M., and Craig, J. B. (1963). Am. J. Ob. Gyn. 85, 105.
Pfeiffer, E., and Davis, G. (1972). J. Am. Geriat. Soc. XX, 151.
Post. F. (1967). The Practitioner 199, 377.
Rahe, H., Mahan, J., Jr., and Arthur, R. J. (1970). J. Psychosomatic Res. 14, 401, 406.
Rhoades, R. P. (1965). Mich. Med. 64, 410.
Rogers, J. (1969). New Engl. J. Med. 280, 264.

Roszak, B. (1969). In "Masculine/Feminine" (B. Roszak, and T. Roszak, eds.), p. 305, Harper and Row Publishing Co., New York.
Rubin, I. (1964). Sexology 30, 709.
Rubin, I. (1966a). In "An Analysis of Human Sexual Response" (R. Brecher, and E. Brecher, eds.), New American Library, New York.
Rubin, I. (1966b). Sexology 32, 512.
Rutherford, R. (1971). Postgrad. Med. 50, 124.
Rutherford, R., and Rutherford, J. (1966). Psychosomatics VII, 89.
Schleyer-Saunders, E. (1971). J. Am. Geriat. Soc. 19, 114.
Scully, D., and Bart, P. (1973). Am. J. Sociol. 78, 1045.
Selye, H. A. (1970). J. Am. Geriat. Soc. XVIII, 669.
Selye, H. A. (1973). Perspectives Biol. Med. 16, 441.
Sheffery, J. B., Wilson, T. A., and Walsh, J. C. (1969). Med. Ann. District Columbia 38, 433.
Shock, N. W. (1970). J. Am. Dietet. Assoc. 56, 491.
Shock, N. W. (1974). In "Theoretical Aspects of Aging" (M. Rockstein, M. L. Sussman, and J. Chesky, eds.), pp. 119-136, Academic Press, New York.
Sontag, S. (1972). Saturday Rev. 55, 29.
Tarail, M. (1962). Sexology 28, 440.
Trimmer, E. J. (1970). "Rejuvenation". A. S. Barnes and Company, New York.
Townsend, C. (1971). "Old Age: The Last Segregation". Grossman Publishers, New York.
Weiss, H. D. (1972). Am. Intern. Med. 76, 793.
Weiss, J. M. (1972). Sci. Am. 226, 104.

EPILOGUE

Ralph Goldman, M.D.

Professor of Medicine and Geriatrics
University of California, Los Angeles
School of Medicine
Los Angeles, California

If the assumption is made that death is due entirely to environmental injury and the individual can be completely protected from the environment, death should be preventable. Accordingly, group survival would conform to curve A in figure 1, and there would be no deaths. This is unlikely, since, in general, fatal events would be random, would tend to be relatively constant over a period of time, and survival should show the pattern in curve B of figure 1. That curve shows a high-risk environment in which 50% of the population dies in each unit of time. At the end of the first unit there would be 50% survivors, at the end of the second unit 25% (50% of 50%), at the end of the third unit 12.5% (50% of 25%), and so forth. The larger the initial population, the longer the survival of the last individual, with (theoretically) infinite survival of an infinitely large cohort. Curve C of figure 1 shows a similar situation in which the mortality has been reduced to 10% per unit of time. In this less rigorous environment, the rate of death would be decreased, median survival would be longer, and cohort survival significantly lengthened. In these patterns, the curves of survival are upwardly concave, downwardly convex.

If, on the other hand, natural death is an internally programmed event and all individuals of a species were identical in this respect, the pattern would conform to curve D of figure 1, and all individuals would die at the same age. Since individuals are not identical, and can be expected to demonstrate a range, a more reasonable pattern might show a distribution (curve E of figure 1).

Early development may be defective and, even if the mature individual is "perfect", the infant and juvenile may not yet be able to withstand the environment, so there may be an excess of early deaths. If this modification is combined with that of curve B in figure 1, another pattern, curve F of figure 1, would be demonstrated. A similar phenomenon, curve G of figure 1, would result in the combination pattern as seen in curve E of figure 1.

Finally, there may be a combination of all three possibilities: early developmental loss, mid-period environmental loss and terminal programmed loss would reveal the pattern seen in curve H of figure 1. This three-component curve should show a downward convexity initially, followed by a sigmoid shape with initial upward convexity in the terminal portion.

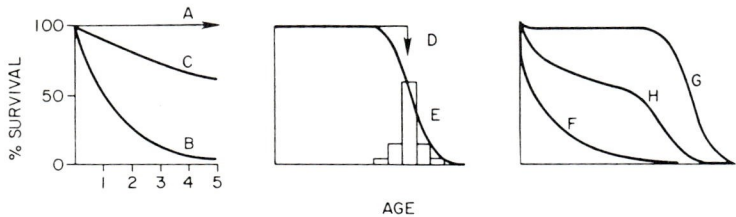

Fig. 1 Possible patterns of cohort survival.

Actual cohort survival curves for various historical periods are shown in figure 2. The bottom curve was plotted for women of the city of York, England, in the 16th century (Cowgill, 1970). There is clearly a large mortality in the first year, followed by an approximately 50% loss every 20 years thereafter (45% one year, 18% twenty year, 11% forty year, and 4% sixty-five year survival). This curve conforms to the concept of severe environmental stress, including an excessive early mortality. There is evidence that at this level of stress the population could not be maintained by the usual human fertility rates, and there must have been a continuous influx of migrants from the countryside.

The next curve is that for English aristocrats of the same period (Cowgill, 1970). This pattern conforms to curve H of figure 1 in which three phases are apparent. Modifications of this configuration are seen in a variety of animal and pre-modern human societies. The exact level of the curve determines the local growth or extinction of a species. All three phases, early developmental defect, intermediate stress, and programmed death are apparent.

The third curve from the bottom is a modified form of the second, and represents the survival of white women in the

United States in 1900 (Anonymous, 1972). The top curve is derived from data on white American women in 1969 (Anonymous, 1972). There is a small initial drop, followed by a very gradually accelerating loss which becomes pronounced in the eighth decade. There is now a more than 96% survival to age 40, 82% to age 65, and 62% to age 75. The evidence for the upwardly concave mid-curve representing random accidental deaths is absent. This curve approaches that of curve G in figure 1, with a small early excess loss and programmed late loss.

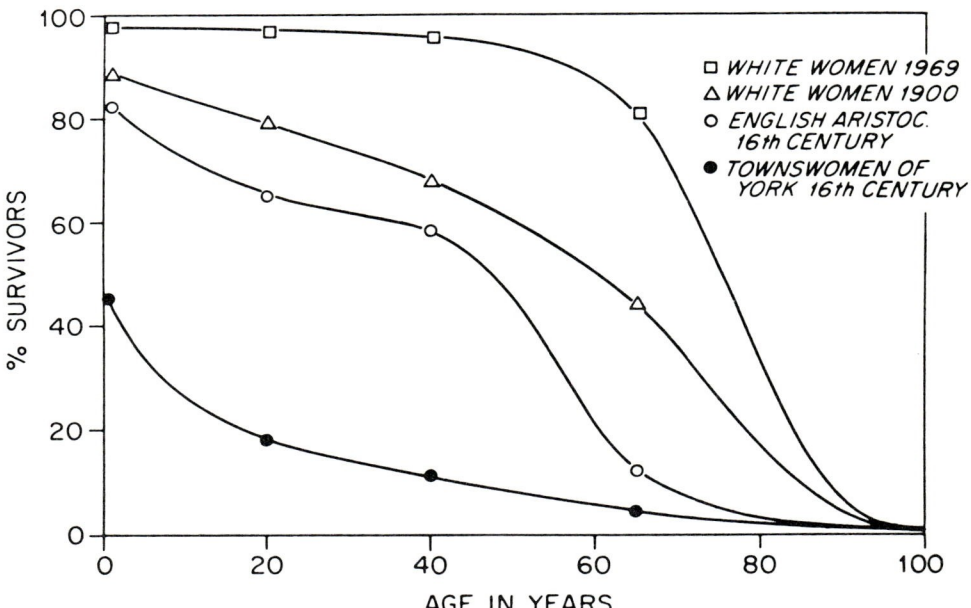

Fig. 2 Actual patterns of cohort survival. Points of origin at the left represent survival at one year.

If these assumptions are essentially correct, a number of important implications can be drawn. Several of these are particularly relevant. It would appear that the extrinsic or environmental causes of death have been largely eliminated in developed societies and that the intrinsic or chiefly constitutional factors are now predominant. It is not argued that because they are constitutional they are not modifiable by environmental factors, but it is probable that these factors operate throughout most of life and that they, in fact, modify the basic constitutional pattern only to a limited extent. These observations explain the slowing down of the improvements in life expectation, despite the recent explosion of basic science knowledge and practical technical application. They also emphasize the central importance of understanding the fundamental nature of the aging process. Clearly, if there is an intrinsic limit to longevity even when all external causes of death are eliminated, further life prolongation will depend upon a modification of the factors which control this limit.

Much social planning for health services is based on the assumption that there is a wide gap between theory and practice. Except for specific populations, the expectations exceed the potential. Public support for service should not obscure the continuing fact that research, such as presented at this meeting, is a relatively small, but essential investment in the continuing search for life prolongation.

REFERENCES

Anonymous (1972). "Statistical Abstract of the United States". United States Government Printing Office, Washington, D. C.

Cowgill, U. M. (1970). Sci. Am. 222, 104.

WITHDRAWN
UST
Libraries